Occlusion: Principles & Treatment

OCCLUSION
Principles & Treatment

José dos Santos, Jr, DDS, PhD

São Paulo, Brazil

Former Professor
Division of Occlusion
Department of Restorative Dentistry
University of Texas Health Science Center at San Antonio
San Antonio, Texas

Quintessence Publishing Co, Inc

Chicago, Berlin, Tokyo, London, Paris, Milan, Barcelona,
Istanbul, São Paulo, Mumbai, Moscow, Prague, and Warsaw

Library of Congress Cataloging-in-Publication Data

Santos Júnior, José dos.
  Occlusion : principles and treatment / Jose dos Santos Jr.
      p. ; cm.
  Includes bibliographical references and index.
  ISBN 978-0-86715-473-3 (hardcover)
  1. Occlusion (Dentistry) 2. Malocclusion—Treatment. I. Title.
  [DNLM: 1. Dental Occlusion. 2. Malocclusion—therapy. 3. Craniomandibular
Disorders—therapy. WU 440 S237o 2007]
  RK523.S34 2007
  617.6'43—dc22

                                                    2007026726

© 2007 Quintessence Publishing Co, Inc

Quintessence Publishing Co, Inc
4350 Chandler Drive
Hanover Park, IL 60133
www.quintpub.com

Editor: Kathryn Funk
Design: Dawn Hartman
Production: Sue Robinson

Printed in Canada

TABLE OF CONTENTS

PREFACE

For many years, it was thought that a single tooth could be the cause of or the solution to all masticatory problems. Such overestimation of the complexity of occlusion created many distortions in treatment planning; in particular, it kept many clinicians from applying occlusal principles to the treatment of temporomandibular disorders. On the other hand, oversimplification of this branch of dental science and its relegation to a secondary role are equally grave mistakes.

All facets of dental treatment require a multidisciplinary approach. According to chaos theory, to understand the fractal dimension of a biologic event, the observer must give substantial attention to every factor. This applies to the behavior of the masticatory system in the sense that every single element of the masticatory apparatus has a role in the occlusal process, as well as in other activities of the craniofacial complex, regardless of the perspective of the observer.

The masticatory apparatus is unique in the human body. The mandible is a very mobile bone within which the dominating functional elements reside: the teeth, alveolar processes, condyles, and attached muscles. It relates to the maxilla, a fixed structure, via teeth in the opposing arches, which contact during mastication. Muscles and a complex neurovascular network are integral to the efficient functioning of the mandible not only in mastication, but also in the proprioceptive control of spatial positions of the jaws, breathing, speech, and swallowing. Consequently, synchronism among the elements of this system during action is critical; what occurs on one side of the mouth must be compensated for on the other side. Therefore, an attentive clinician must keep the interocclusal relationship of a patient under constant observation during treatment of the masticatory system.

Literature on the subject of occlusion is extensive, varied, and confusing, giving rise to a great deal of controversy. Many theories have been advanced to explain and guide professionals in the use of techniques and clinical approaches, seeking varied objectives. Some theories are now outmoded because of their limited goals and dated observations, while others have produced rational methods of treatment. Nonetheless, their application requires a balanced and accurate understanding of the science of occlusion. It is my sincere hope that this introduction to the principles and treatment of occlusion will lead professionals to review and apply the different schools of thought within the science of occlusion in a critical manner.

MAXILLOMANDIBULAR RELATIONS AND MOVEMENTS

The topic of dental occlusion tends to generate many discussions.[1-9] Several theories have been proposed, but all of them are either poorly understood or insufficiently elaborated to substantiate prevailing ideologies. Consensus in this area will always be difficult to achieve, because specific explanations will always rely on the scientific and clinical foundations of the individuals interested in this subject. This longstanding conflict has involved several disciplines, and, not surprisingly, each dental specialty bases its theories on observations made from its own clinical perspective. Consequently, dental clinicians find it difficult to synthesize the information and apply it to the treatment of patients,[10-18] particularly those who present with functional problems of the masticatory apparatus.

Maxillomandibular functional relationships have two distinct movement patterns: one involves contact between occlusal surfaces during sliding motions, and the other involves contact-free opening and closing of the mandible.

Examination of tooth contacts between opposing occlusal surfaces discloses many variations.[19-24] These contacts may be viewed as either centric positions or eccentric movements. To determine the occluding action between opposing arches, it is necessary to analyze tooth contact during functional (chewing) action. Parafunctional contacts may be found in some patients as well. This chapter describes centric positions and eccentric movements, as well as the noncontacting relationship at rest (or postural) position, which influences mandibular dynamics.

CENTRIC POSITIONS

Centric describes tooth contacts made between centric jaw relation and maximum intercuspation. These two positions have been the subject of a number of clinical and theoretical controversies. Demands for scientific evidence have led to studies that allowed a better understanding of the significance of these positions.[1-4] Occlusal adjustment procedures and oral rehabilitations use centric position as the basis for developing an occlusal scheme.

Maximum intercuspation

The maxillomandibular position termed *maximum intercuspation* (also known as *centric occlusion, habitual centric, acquired centric, intercuspation position,* and *power centric*) represents the intercuspation of opposing occlusal surfaces, the stage at which the mastication cycle is initiated (Fig 1-1). The proprioceptive sense of this interocclusal relationship is developed during infancy. It originates as a reflex arch, which is then permanently imprinted in higher centers of the nervous system and controls the servomechanism of the masticatory function. One hypothesis is that this relationship encourages maximum contraction of masticatory muscle forces to develop.[19,25]

Physiologically, centric occlusion might be a specific stage of mandibular function; however, numerous clinical conditions such as occlusal problems, muscular symptoms, and temporomandibular joint (TMJ) changes can produce deviations from this norm.[26] This position is also highly affected by head posture: Bringing the head forward from the upward position or stretching it backward will produce different initial centric occlusal contacts. Therefore, because clinical reproducibility of the intercuspation position is in doubt, it is not advisable to use centric occlusion as a reference for mounting casts on an articulator during comprehensive rehabilitations.

Maximum intercuspation position is closely related to the curve of Spee (also known as the *curve of occlusion* or *compensation curve*) because the vertical dimension of occlusion depends on the plane of occlusion (Fig 1-2). Because of the limitations imposed by the curve of Spee, it is unwise to lengthen clinical crowns during occlusal rehabilitation.

During intercuspation, the condyles place limited stress on their respective articular surfaces (Fig 1-3). Because centric occlusion is viewed as a physiologic position, chewing strokes always begin and conclude at the centric contacts.

Centric relation

Distinct from maximum intercuspation, which is a muscular position, *centric relation* is believed to be a ligamentous position. Centric relation is a position where the hinge movement of the mandible (known as the *terminal hinge axis*) can take place. In clinical practice, this hinge axis determination is valuable because it is reproducible. When comprehensive occlusal rehabilitation is contemplated for a patient who has lost a great deal of occlusal surface substance, this reproducibility is important because dental casts are related to each other on the articulator according to the hinge axis (Fig 1-4). In the absence of maximum intercuspal position in edentulous patients, patients with loose teeth, and patients with other types of lost occlusal relationships, centric relation is used to fabricate a prosthetic reconstruction.

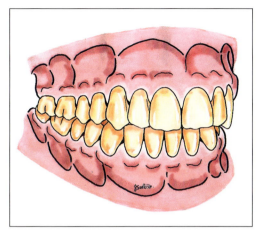

Fig 1-1 Occlusal relationship in maximum intercuspation in habitual jaw position.

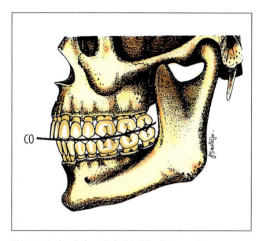

Fig 1-2 Occlusal plane *(solid black line)*. Curve of Spee or curve of occlusion (CO).

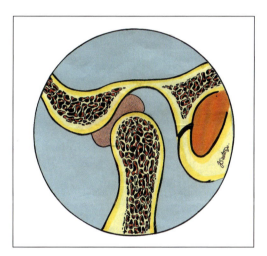

Fig 1-3 Relationship between the condyle and glenoid fossa when the teeth are in maximum intercuspation.

A classic example of the controversial nature of the concept of occlusion concerns the position of the mandible in centric relation. Many scientific articles offer definitions of this position, and even the *Glossary of Prosthodontics Terms*[27] reports several different descriptions of this key mandibular location. It is important to emphasize that centric relation is as personal as an individual's fingerprint; when the mandible is guided to centric relation, the condylar position varies according to its anatomy as well as the morphology of the glenoid fossa. This relationship is also conditional on the integrity of the joints and related structures.

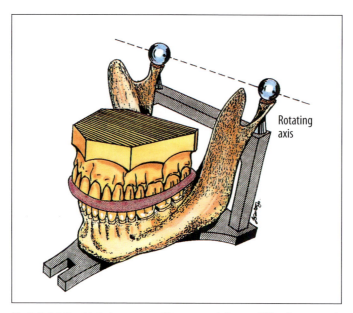

Fig 1-4 Relationship between a maxillary cast and the mandible when a centric relation bite registration is used to mount a cast in the articulator, according to a rotating or epicenter axis.

It has been theorized that, in centric relation, the mandible rotates around a single axis passing through both condyles to produce a hinge movement (Fig 1-5). However, it is unlikely that, when the jaw is manipulated into a hinge position, the axis of rotation will traverse the center of both condyles simultaneously. More likely, this spinning movement generates an instantaneous axis of rotation that, in many cases, is disengaged off the condyles and may be correlated to the anterior eminence of the articular surfaces according to a superior, posterior, or anterior location. Clinically, the most accurate description of the axis of rotation would be that the condylar heads are in the uppermost, midmost, and rearmost locations in their glenoid fossae (Fig 1-6). Studies support that this position is the most superior position of the condyle rather than the most retruded position.[4,5,14,18] Thus, the posture assumed by the condyles in centric relation has little bearing in capturing the hinge movement. For the dental practitioner, what is critical is to direct the mandible in a consistent and replicating pivot movement without applying stress to the joints and adjacent structures.

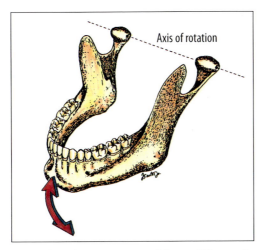

Fig 1-5 *(arrow)* Hinge movement of the mandible around a common horizontal axis.

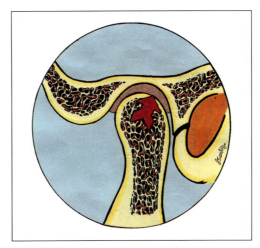

Fig 1-6 Relationship between the condyle and glenoid fossa when the jaw is in centric relation. *(arrow)* Orientation of the condyle within the joint (usually uppermost and rearmost position).

REST POSITION

The *rest position* of the mandible has elicited many discussions and much dispute (Fig 1-7).[8,13,14,26] Despite scientific advances in the fields of electromyography, cinefluorography, radiology, laminography, tomography, computed tomography, magnetic resonance, and kinesiology, few theories about this posture have been advanced. Considering the complex neuromuscular activation of the masticatory system, it may be more accurate to characterize this position as *postural*. The posture of the mandible can encompass the equilibrium of the elevator and depressor masticatory muscles as well as their viscoelastic qualities. These conditions keep the mandible suspended at a particular interocclusal distance, also known as the *interocclusal rest space* (Fig 1-8). Most experts calculate the interocclusal rest space to be between 1 and 3 mm. The space must be maintained; it may neither be augmented to produce infraocclusion nor reduced to produce supraocclusion during rehabilitation procedures.[28]

It is possible that, at this mandibular location, muscle fibers are at their optimal extent with a minimal volley of neural impulses. From this stage, muscles can readily initiate either elevation or depression of the mandible. It appears that, from this position, masticatory muscles may start contraction to achieve the maximum possible force that will produce total intercuspation.

The rest position of the mandible is relatively constant even throughout some movements of the body. However, the posture of the head can momentarily alter the space between opposing occlusal surfaces. For example, flexing the head

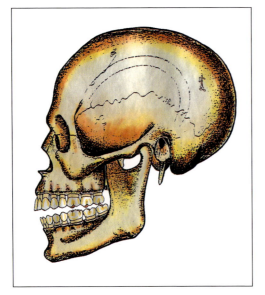

Fig 1-7 Mandible in rest position.

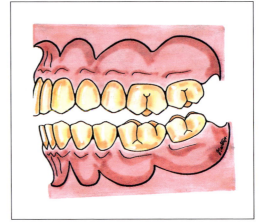

Fig 1-8 Interocclusal rest space.

backward will change this relationship and develop a greater space. Conversely, bending the head forward will bring the maxilla and mandible toward each other, and the teeth will sometimes come into contact, entirely eliminating the interocclusal rest space. Loss of teeth and emotional conditions (eg, anxiety) related to habits such as bruxism and clenching can adversely affect the rest position.

ECCENTRIC POSITIONS

All movements of the mandible can be traced in three dimensions and are best evaluated when projected and viewed in orthogonal spatial planes. These projections and registrations document *border movements* of the mandible beyond which movement is not possible. Such movements are reproducible. Within these limits *functional movements* are developed, which unlike border movements are not reproducible. Recordings of these limits sometimes make it possible to assess the influences of mandibular movements in the diagnosis and analysis of occlusal equilibrium.

Because orthogonal planes intersect each other perpendicularly (forming 90-degree angles), it is possible to isolate just three planes that are valuable for the study of mandibular movements (Fig 1-9):

Fig 1-9 Orthogonal planes of reference in relation to the head: frontal or coronal plane, horizontal plane, and sagittal plane.

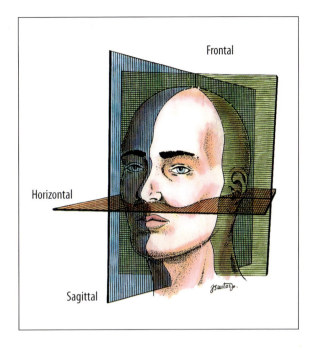

1. Sagittal plane: Bisects the skull into two symmetric mirror images oriented anteroposteriorly.
2. Frontal or coronal plane: Positioned toward the face and oriented practically parallel to the labial surface of the incisors. Always perpendicular to the horizontal and sagittal planes, this plane may be moved anteroposteriorly to intersect the head at different points. In Fig 1-9 it is positioned at the TMJs.
3. Horizontal plane: Parallel to the floor. This plane may be moved superiorly or inferiorly.

Border movements in relation to the sagittal plane

When recorded at the anterior teeth, mandibular border movements generate a characteristic diagram known as the *Posselt diagram* (Figs 1-10 and 1-11), which reflects the movement of the TMJs (Fig 1-12). Distinct from pantographic tracings of mandibular movement, the Posselt diagram embodies a sideways projection of the envelope of motion. Segments of this motion are inscribed during tooth contact and depression and elevation of the mandible. During tooth contact, it is possible to observe maximum intercuspation (Fig 1-13), centric relation positions (Figs 1-14 and 1-15), edge-to-edge occlusion (Fig 1-16), postural or rest position (Fig 1-17), and maximum protrusion (Fig 1-18). Direct measurement of these positions in the patient is described at the end of this chapter.

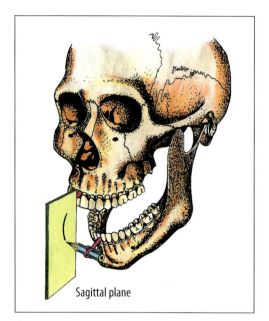

Fig 1-10 Inscribing pencil in relation to the sagittal plane when the Posselt diagram is recorded.

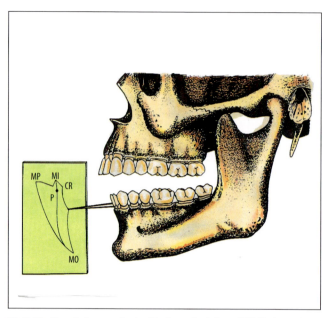

Fig 1-11 Posselt diagram obtained in the sagittal plane. (MI) Maximum intercuspation (centric occlusion); (CR) centric relation contact; (MO) maximum opening; (MP) maximum protrusion; (P) postural or rest position.

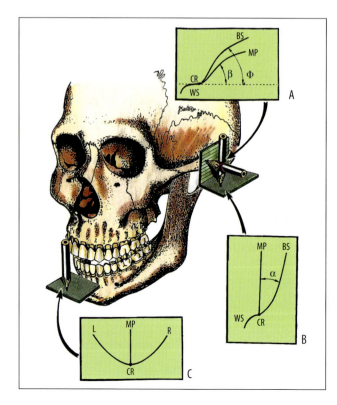

Fig 1-12 Gnathologic pantograph. (A) Sagittal plane at the temporomandibular joint. The lines represent the movements of the inscribing pencil when moving from centric relation (CR) to maximum protrusion (MP) and from centric relation (CR) to balancing side (BS). The path inscribed by the condyle in working-side (WS) movement is also shown. Angle β represents condylar guidance. Angle Φ represents the Fischer angle. (B) Horizontal plane at the temporomandibular joint. Movements starting from centric relation (CR) to maximum protrusion (MP) and from centric relation (CR) to balancing side (BS) are shown. The working-side (WS) movement is also shown. Angle α measures the Bennett angle. (C) Horizontal plane, illustrating the movement of the anterior portion of the dentition. The pencil records the movement from centric relation (CR) to maximum protrusion (MP) and the lateral movements from centric relation to the left (L) and right (R) sides.

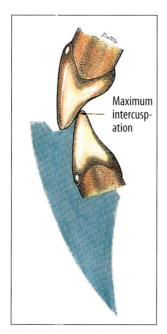

Fig 1-13 Maximum intercuspation contact (centric occlusion) at the incisors.

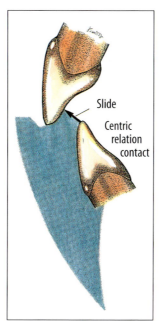

Fig 1-14 Centric relation contact relationship at the incisors.

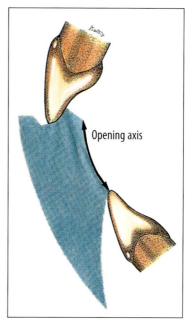

Fig 1-15 Arc produced during hinge opening of the mandible, as observed at the incisors.

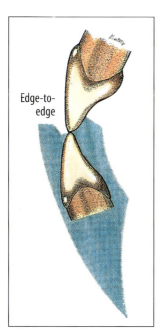

Fig 1-16 Edge-to-edge relationship between incisors.

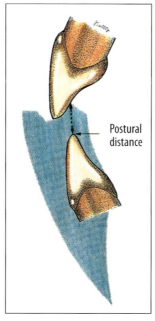

Fig 1-17 Measurement of the distance between opposing incisors in the rest (postural) position.

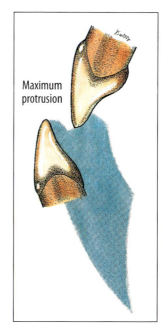

Fig 1-18 Maximum protrusion at the incisors.

Rotation and translation of condyles

Condylar rotation and translation are part of the border movements; although not markedly visible during mandibular functional chewing movements, they can easily be seen when viewed in the sagittal plane.

When the mandible is guided to centric relation, opposing teeth present first contact relationship (Fig 1-19), or even a slip from *centric relation occlusion* (or the first point of contact in centric relation) to maximum intercuspation. This is an indication that the condyles are located in the uppermost and rearmost position in the glenoid fossa. The beginning of mandibular movement can be an arc opening of approximately 2.5 cm between opposing incisors (Fig 1-20). This arc opening is assumed to produce simultaneous rotation of both condyles around a secure and clinically reproducible hinge axis. This purely hinge movement is known as *terminal hinge movement*. The term *terminal* implies that when the mandible is made to produce the first tooth contact in centric relation occlusion, and the subject tightens the masticatory muscles, a slide toward maximum intercuspation is produced (Fig 1-21). This will be the last movement before coming into maximum intercuspation. The recording of the terminal hinge axis and first contact in centric relation are visible in the posterior portion of the Posselt diagram.

An increase of arc opening around the terminal hinge will produce translational movement of the condyles against the articular eminence. The translational movement from this position produces a curved pathway that terminates in maximum opening of the jaw (Figs 1-22 and 1-23).

From maximum intercuspation, the subject can thrust the mandible forward, reaching full protrusion (Figs 1-24 and 1-25). The Posselt diagram now displays the position of the incisive point located at the anterior limit or border position of the mandible, with the teeth in contact.

From maximum protrusion, the mandible can be hinged to reach a position of maximum opening.

Mandibular protraction

Inaccurate interpretation of some terms used in the international vocabulary, specifically terms derived from the English language, has produced a great deal of disagreement among dental professionals. An example of this confusion is related to the expression *mandibular protraction*, used to describe the activation of the medial pterygoid muscle, which should not be confused with *mandibular protrusion*. During chewing, the mobilization of the medial pterygoid muscle for mandibular elevation produces simultaneously an abrupt anterior translational movement of the jaw to adapt to the bolus of food. Because *protractor* is a term utilized to designate the instrument for angular measurement, by extension *protraction of the mandible* in this instance may suggest angular projection of

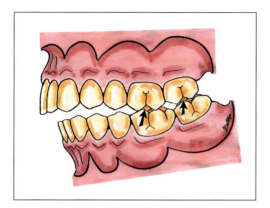

Fig 1-19 First centric relation contact in lateral view. Note the molar relationships where the first contacts occur between the occlusal inclines *(arrows)*.

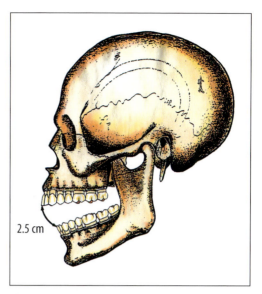

Fig 1-20 Hinge opening around a transverse axis. The rotation around the axis produces limited opening of the jaw (2.5 cm).

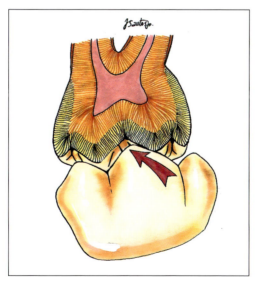

Fig 1-21 Direction of the centric slide *(arrow)*, starting from an unstable position in centric relation to maximum intercuspation.

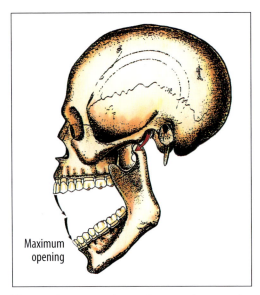

Fig 1-22 A more extensive opening, to maximum opening of the jaw, is made in two stages *(arrows)*. The condyles rotate and translate simultaneously.

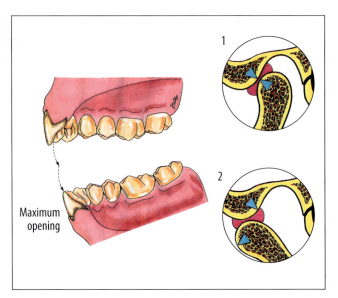

Fig 1-23 During maximum opening of the jaw, the condyle moves from (1) a centered position in the temporomandibular joint to (2) an extreme displacement of the condyle. The displacement of the *blue arrowheads* reveals the tendency for simultaneous translation and rotation of the condyle in the joint. The incisor relationship indicates mandibular movement *(black arrows)* to maximum opening.

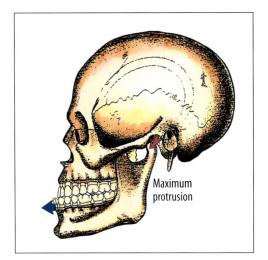

Fig 1-24 Full anterior thrust *(blue arrow)* of the mandible in protrusive movement. In this case, maximum translation of the condyles *(red arrow)* occurs with minimal rotation.

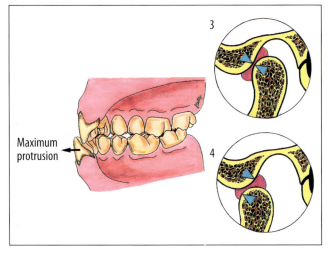

Fig 1-25 During maximum protrusive movement, the condyles move from (3) a centered position to (4) an anterior position. There is translation *(blue arrowheads)* and almost no rotation of condyles. Note the effect on the relationships at the anterior teeth *(black arrow)*.

mandibular movement. A single word probably cannot accurately define this action. Other examples may be encountered in the dental literature where the syntax used does not conform to the scientific perspective.

Inside the limits of the Posselt diagram, which represents border movements of the mandible, the mandible may assume an infinite number of positions, the most notable of which is related to the resting or postural position.

Border movements in relation to the frontal or coronal plane

Registration of border movements related to the frontal or coronal plane can be viewed both at the incisors and TMJs. For didactic purposes, it is best to start from maximum intercuspation (Fig 1-26).

Eccentric movements of the mandible, when observed at the level of the joints, present different characteristics depending on the side to which the mandible moves. If the mandible slides to the left, the left condyle tends to remain inside the articular fossa, also presenting a rotational movement. This condyle (in this case the left one) is then called the *rotating condyle* or *working condyle*. The right condyle in left movement translates forward, inward, and downward along the articular eminence. This right condyle is then identified as the *translating condyle* or *balancing condyle* (Fig 1-27). If the mandible slides to the right side, the situation is reversed.

When the eccentric movements are observed at the anterior teeth, the mandible scribes lines of lateral movements to the right and left (Fig 1-28). A subject can depress the jaw from centric occlusion to maximum opening, producing a vertical line. If the mandible is depressed from a lateral position, the result is a curved path ending at maximum opening (see Fig 1-28). At the joints, to achieve maximum opening of the jaw, the left condyle must also translate forward at the same time. As the maximum limit of mandibular opening is reached, there can be no lateral movement. From this maximum opening, the subject can move the jaw to the left lateral position. In doing so, the left condyle must translate backward while the right condyle is kept in forward position. The chewing cycle and speaking are considered intraborder movements, and when viewed from the frontal plane, at the dentition, these movements produce a teardrop shape (Fig 1-29).

Bennett movement or shift

The condyles do not have a perfectly spherical configuration, and similarly the articular fossae and eminences are not perfectly concave. In addition, factors

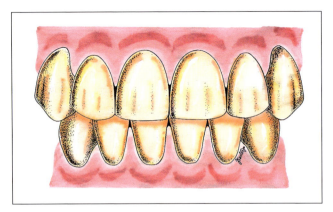

Fig 1-26   Maximum intercuspation.

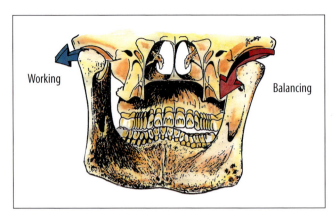

Fig 1-27   Left working movement as viewed from the back of the skull (frontal plane). Note the translation *(red arrow)* of the right balancing condyle and the lateral shift *(blue arrow)* of the left working condyle.

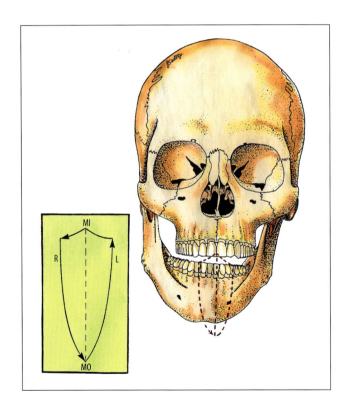

Fig 1-28   Border movements recorded in the frontal plane. (MI) Maximum intercuspation (centric occlusion); (R) right lateral movement; (L) left lateral movement; (MO) maximum opening.

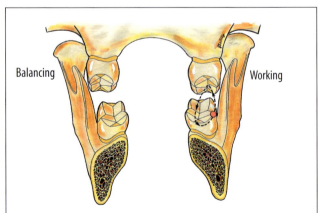

Fig 1-29   Frontal view of the path *(arrows)* developed during a left-side chewing cycle. The tip of the supporting cusp of the mandibular molar *(red dot)* is producing the functional movement in relation to the central fossa of the maxillary molar.

Fig 1-30 Two types of lateral eccentric movement *(red arrow)* to the left working side. One is performed without Bennett movement and has limited displacement *(blue dots)*. The other, performed with Bennett movement, presents a more extensive lateral displacement *(red dots)*.

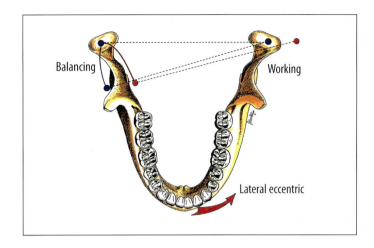

such as contraction of some mastication muscles attached to the condyle and disk, restraint of ligaments in joints, warping of the mandible, etc, all contribute to prevent purely rotational and translational movements of the mandible. Therefore, during lateral movements, especially when observed on the frontal plane, there is no pure rotation and translation of condyles in their joints. There is a tendency for a shift of the jaw toward the side to which the mandible is moving. This lateral bodily displacement of the mandible, known as the *Bennett movement* or the *Bennett shift*, may be absent or obvious in different subjects (Fig 1-30). The importance of this fact is related to the pathways across which maxillary and mandibular opposing occlusal surface cusps are supposed to glide during functional eccentric movements.

Border movements in relation to the horizontal plane

Mandibular motions projected on the horizontal plane can also be analyzed at both the incisors and temporomandibular joints. The respective tracks represent distinct outlines for each position or registration. Movements recorded at the dentition have concurrent translations of one or both condyles.

The following example would result if a pencil were attached to the anterior portion of the maxilla and kept in contact with a flat and horizontally oriented plate attached to the mandibular incisors (Fig 1-31). With the opposing teeth almost in contact, the mandible produces a right lateral movement, without Bennett shift. The left condyle translates and the right condyle only has a tendency to rotate, producing a slightly curved lateral path on the recording plate (Fig 1-32).

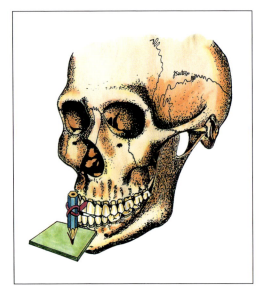

Fig 1-31 Position of the horizontal plane and inscribing pencil for recording of border movements.

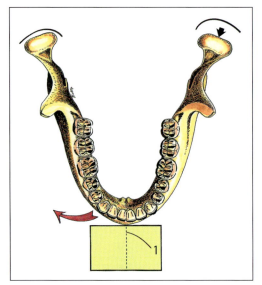

Fig 1-32 Border movements recorded on the horizontal plane. (1) First stage of the movement from maximum intercuspation. The left condyle translates forward *(arrowhead)*. The mandible performs a right lateral movement *(red arrow)*. The inscribing plane is attached to the mandible.

From this initial position, the right condyle is now made to translate forward. The mandible moves to maximum protrusion and the pencil has scribed a second path (Fig 1-33). It is important to note that in full protrusion both condyles translate forward, and in lateral eccentric movement just one condyle translates.

Next, the left condyle retracts, producing a left lateral movement of the jaw. The pencil scribes a lateral path on the plate in the opposite direction from the previous path (Fig 1-34). To complete this cycle of movement, the left condyle remains practically stationary and the right condyle is now translated backward. The pencil will trace the corresponding path for the movement (Fig 1-35). The final result of this cycle will be a diamond-shaped diagram on the tracing plate. This diamond diagram embodies the outer limit of mandibular movements inside which the mandible is free to move. The sides of the diamond are considered clinically reproducible positions.

If the aforementioned movements start from centric relation instead of maximum intercuspation, the posterior corner of the diagram, corresponding to centric relation position, represents an important clinical landmark for rehabilitation procedures, especially involving complete-denture construction. Tracings originating from centric relation are commonly called *Gothic arch tracings* or *arrow point tracings* (Fig 1-36).

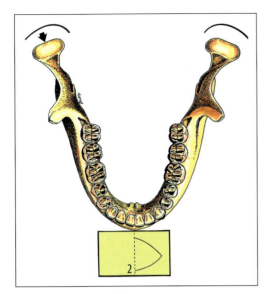

Fig 1-33 (2) Stage 2 of the recording. The right condyle translates forward *(arrowhead)*. The mandible now goes to maximum protrusion.

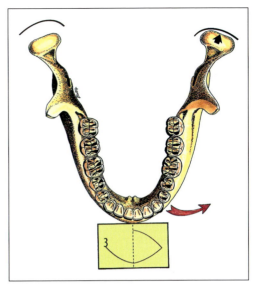

Fig 1-34 (3) Stage 3 of the recording. The left condyle retracts *(arrowhead)*. The mandible now performs a left lateral movement *(red arrow)*.

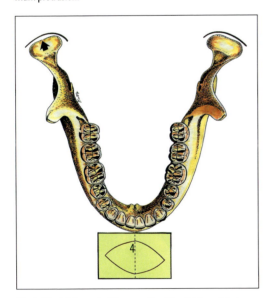

Fig 1-35 (4) Stage 4 of the recording. The right condyle translates backward *(arrowhead)*. The mandible returns to maximum intercuspation.

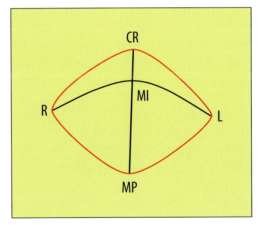

Fig 1-36 Complete record of border movements on the horizontal plane. (CR) Centric relation; (MI) maximum intercuspation; (MP) maximum protrusion; (R) right lateral movement; (L) left lateral movement.

Fischer angle

A disputable aspect in occlusion is associated with the Fischer angle. The trajectory that produces the Fischer angle represents the measurement of the lateral displacement of the balancing condyle, which is projected on the sagittal or frontal planes (taking as reference a horizontal line).

The pathway delineated by the condyle on the summit of the glenoid fossa creates simultaneous three-dimensional trajectories as related to orthogonal planes in space (Fig 1-37). These movements may be recorded as forward, downward, and medial translation. The translational movement of the balancing condyle, originating in centric position (ie, centric occlusion or centric relation), may be particularly recorded on the sagittal and frontal cranial planes of reference. Because the Fischer angle includes part of the condylar action in three dimensions, it records part of the mandibular track conformed to the frontal plane. Indeed, for better discernment, the path that produces the Fischer angle is best regarded in relation to an anterior-posterior or posterior-anterior inspection of the skull.

The Fischer angle is normally assessed on sagittal projections according to a horizontal line. However, the trajectory that defines this angle is independent of the condylar path that measures condylar guidance.

If the trajectory that defines the Fischer angle is inscribed on the horizontal plane, it may concur with the so-called pathway of the Bennett angle. The pathway that defines the Bennett angle has profound implications in the determination of the Fischer angle. This translational movement is not depicted as a straight line; it is typically described according to a curved path, which comprises two stages: immediate lateral movement and progressive lateral movement. The immediate lateral movement (known as *side shift*) may be arched downward and, when projected on the frontal plane, encompasses part of the Fischer angle. When the trajectory generating the Fischer angle is flat, taking as reference the horizontal line (ie, without any downward and medial inclination), the angular value is zero. It is essential to estimate the length of the sideways movement of the condyle without any downward or medial translation; a lengthy sideways movement, for example, would be the probable result of ineffective canine guidance.

Three-dimensional envelope of motion

All the details of movements projected on three-dimensional planes deliver practical value during analysis of the occlusal determinants as influenced by mandibular dynamics. It is possible to create a characteristic framework from compositions of movements at the anterior teeth, using simultaneous projections recorded on the orthogonal planes (Fig 1-38). If a solid based on this framework is constructed,

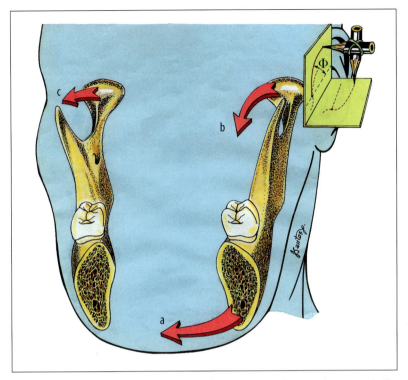

Fig 1-37 Measurement of the Fischer angle (Φ) in relation to the sagittal pantograph. The mandible is producing a right working movement *(arrow a)*. The path of the left balancing condyle *(arrow b)* produces the sagittal recording simultaneously with the horizontal recording. The right working condyle exhibits a lateral displacement *(arrow c)*.

the result will be an *envelope of motion* containing the outer limits of mandibular border movements (Fig 1-39). In Figs 1-39 and 1-40, the horizontal diamond-shaped diagram is formed at different levels of mandibular opening, and the horizontal diagrams grow smaller as they approach maximum opening. At maximum opening, projection on the orthogonal planes forms a point from which no movements are possible.

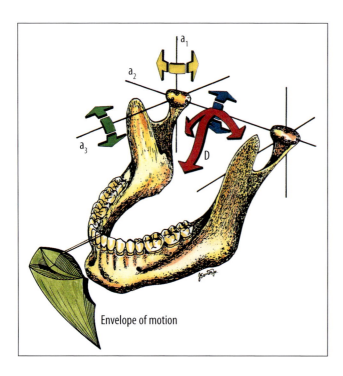

Envelope of motion

Fig 1-38 Movements of the mandible as determined by the envelope of motion generated at the anterior portion of the jaw. Condylar rotation and translation around vertical (a₁) *(yellow arrows)*, horizontal (a₂) *(blue arrows)*, and lateral (a₃) *(green arrows)* axes. (D) Displacement of the mandible *(red arrows)* in protrusive and eccentric lateral movements.

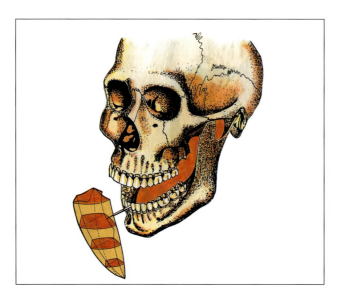

Fig 1-39 Three-dimensional envelope of motion generated at the anterior portion of the mandible.

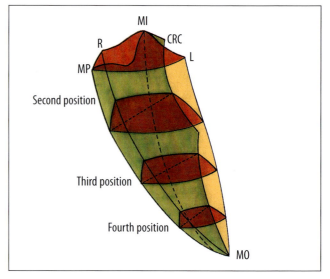

Fig 1-40 Envelope of motion. The more the mandible opens (progressing from second to fourth positions), the less the area covered by the horizontal border movement. In maximum opening (MO), there is no formation of a horizontal diagram. (MI) Maximum intercuspation; (CRC) centric relation contact; (MP) maximum protrusion; (R) right lateral movement; (L) left lateral movement.

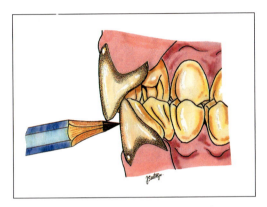

Fig 1-41 Marking of the overbite. This is the first step in assessment of the dimensions of mandibular movements.

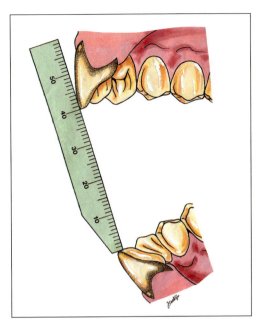

Fig 1-42 Measurement of voluntary mouth opening starting from maximum intercuspation. The total measurement of the maximum opening must include the amount of overbite.

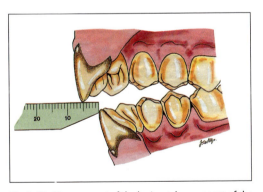

Fig 1-43 Measurement of the horizontal component of the centric relation slide.

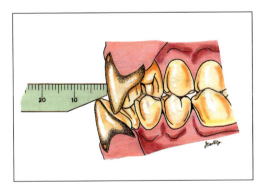

Fig 1-44 Measurement of maximum protrusion.

Measuring the ranges of mandibular movements

Figures 1-41 to 1-46 depict the sequence of procedures for measuring mandibular range of border movements tracking the mesial-incisal-facial point angle of a mandibular central incisor during certain positions and habitual closure.

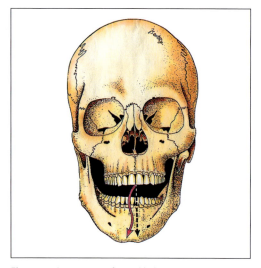

Fig 1-45 Assessment of mandibular movement deviation *(red arrow)* in maximum opening. *Black arrow* represents normal movement.

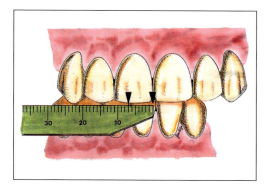

Fig 1-46 Measurement of the right lateral displacement of the mandible. The midlines between the maxillary and mandibular central incisors *(arrowsheads)* are used as reference.

MASTICATION

Mastication[29-31] is a complex activity accomplished by a unique arrangement of the muscles of the head and neck and the maxillomandibular relationship. The mandible has a great deal of mobility, and the teeth, alveolar processes, and condyles are its dominating functional elements. The mandible and mandibular functions are related to the maxilla (a fixed structure), which also contains teeth and alveolar processes.

The movements of the mandible are controlled by muscles and a complex neurovascular network that allows not only mastication but proprioceptive control of the spatial position of the jaws, breathing, speech, swallowing, and other complex activities.[32] It is critical that all parts of the system operate in a synchronized way to function efficiently and effectively. Consequently, depending on the activity, a muscle will be active one moment and inactive the next. Groups of muscles have concurrent (protagonist or synergistic) actions during a given functional movement to promote efficient chewing. Therefore, muscles on one side of the mouth must compensate for muscular activity on the other side.

Although it is difficult to clearly demonstrate the antagonist action of a muscle or group of muscles, the most convincing evidence for this antagonistic activity is the gradual decrease in contractile activity when the opposite muscle or group of muscles becomes active. Balance between contraction and inhibition is developed to prevent sudden, snapping movements of the jaws during functional movements.

The following section describes the interrelationships of the teeth, muscles, and joints during empty movements of the jaws and chewing. A brief anatomic description of masticatory muscles, including detailed explanations of their actions as a group during empty movements of the jaws and during phases of the masticatory process, will follow.

Masticatory muscles

Masseter muscle

Body of the masseter muscle
At its origin, this portion of the muscle has a long tendinous attachment to two thirds of the anterior lower border of the zygomatic arch and lateral surface of the ascending ramus of the mandible; some fibers may be attached to the coronoid process. The insertion of the bulk of its muscular structure is close to the mandibular angle (Fig 1-47).

As a powerful mandibular elevator muscle, this portion of the masseter muscle is readily sensitive to aggressive bruxing habits and joint problems.

The superficial portion of the masseter muscle covers a great part of the deep layer (see Fig 1-47).

Deep layer of the masseter muscle
The most posterior fibers of this muscle present distal divergent orientation in relation to the superficial masseter. The tendinous attachment of this muscle originates on the lower lateral border of the zygomatic arch and lateral surface of the mandibular ramus. The insertion is concurrent with the superficial layer, at the mandibular angle.

This deep layer of the muscle is primarily in charge of the retrusive range of mandible movements and becomes frequently sensitive in the presence of bruxing habits associated with deflective occlusal contacts at centric relation.

Temporalis muscle

Body of the temporalis muscle
The fan-shaped arrangement of the fibers of this muscle attached to the side of the skull may define different functional areas. Therefore, this muscle is usually described as having anterior, middle, and posterior bundles. The origin of the muscle is associated with the temporal bone, temporal fossa, and fascia. The insertion occurs at the coronoid process, and the tendinous attachment may extend to the anterior border of the mandible ramus (Fig 1-48).

The anterior and intermediate bundles of this muscle are partially responsible for mandibular elevation and very sensitive to occlusal interference. The posteri-

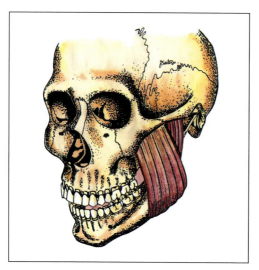

Fig 1-47 Anatomic location of the masseter muscle.

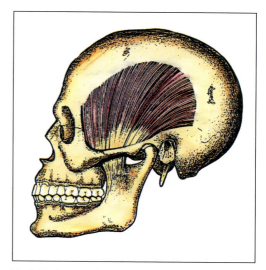

Fig 1-48 Anatomic location of the temporalis muscle.

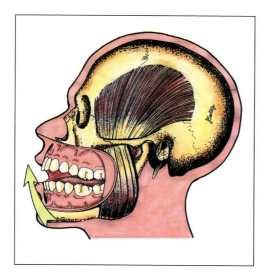

Fig 1-49 Combined action of the masseter and temporalis muscles to elevate the mandible *(arrow)*.

or bundle, due to its horizontal and backward orientation, is responsible for the retrusive action of the mandibular bone.

Insertion of the temporalis muscle

Intraoral access for palpation of the temporalis muscle is related to its tendinous insertion on the coronoid process and anterior border of the mandible (see Fig 1-48).

As a positioner of the mandible, this muscle is usually sensitive to occlusal discrepancies, especially those related to centric and eccentric mandibular positions. The combined action of the masseter and temporalis muscles comprises the most potent function for mandibular elevation (Fig 1-49).

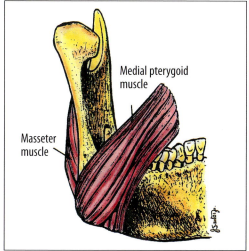
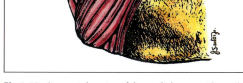

Fig 1-50 Anatomic location of the medial pterygoid muscle.

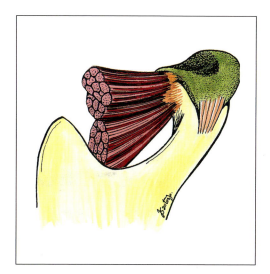

Fig 1-51 Anatomic location of the lateral pterygoid muscle.

Pterygoid muscles

Medial pterygoid muscle

This muscle, internally located in relation to the ascending ramus of the mandible, runs almost parallel to the masseter muscle. The tendinous origin of this muscle is related to the internal surface of the lateral pterygoid plate and pyramidal process of the palatine bone, and some fibers may be attached to the maxillary tuberosity. The insertion of the bulk of the muscle is on the internal surface of the mandibular ramus and angle of the mandible (Fig 1-50).

During mandibular elevation, both medial pterygoid muscles have a combined function (synergistic action); however, each medial pterygoid muscle also assists in lateral excursions of the jaw.

Lateral pterygoid muscle

This muscle[33, 34] is usually described as having two heads (superior and inferior). The origin of the superior head is at the infratemporal portion of the sphenoid great wing. The insertion of its tendinous process is on the anterior border of the condylar disc, on the condylar capsule, and on the neck of the condyle (at the level of the fovea). The origin of the inferior head is at the lateral surface of the pterygoid plate. The insertion of its tendinous portion is mostly related to the condylar capsule and mandible fovea.

Some authors consider these muscles as separate entities[33,34]; however, there is no consensus about this condition, because sometimes these two portions do not function independently (Fig 1-51).

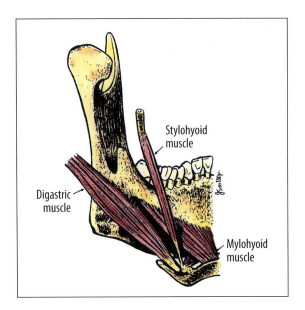

Fig 1-52 Anatomic location of the suprahyoid musculature.

Because there is limited access for intraoral palpation of this muscle, the area corresponding to the location of both lateral pterygoid muscles has been described as the *pterygoid window*. The location of the pterygoid window is represented by a narrow access behind the maxillary tuberosity, in an upward direction.

Limitations of mandibular movements resulting from occlusal prematurities in centric and eccentric interferences may produce increased sensitivity in this group of muscles.

Suprahyoid muscles

Although there are other muscles, the suprahyoid muscles most involved in the depression of the mandible are the digastric, mylohyoid, and stylohyoid muscles.

Digastric muscle

Anterior belly of the digastric muscle. The origin of this muscle is at the digastric fossa in the anterior inner surface of the mandible body. From this origin, the muscle moves in a medial, posterior, and inferior direction, where its tendinous insertion continues with the tendinous insertion of the posterior belly of the digastric muscle on the same side of the head. Both tendons pass through a fibrous loop of the hyoid bone without any apparent attachment to the bone.

Posterior belly of the digastric muscle. The origin of this muscle is at the mastoid notch of the temporal bone. From this origin, the muscle is oriented in a forward, medial, and inferior direction to reach its tendinous insertion with the tendon of the anterior belly of the digastric muscle through the fibrous loop of the hyoid bone (Fig 1-52).

As an important depressor of the mandible, this pair of muscles may be sensitive to some forms of dysfunction involving the temporomandibular joint.

Mylohyoid muscle
This muscle, existing in pairs, is attached, side-to-side, to a median raphe from the chin to the hyoid bone. The origin of the muscle, on each side, is at the mylohyoid line in the inner surface of the mandible. This pair of muscles spreads from the last molar to the mandibular symphysis. From the origin, each pair of muscles is oriented in a medial and inferior direction to attach on the upper surface of the hyoid bone (see Fig 1-52).

These muscles elevate the hyoid bone, base of the tongue, and floor of the mouth. They assist in the depression of the mandible when the hyoid bone is stabilized.

Stylohyoid muscle
The origin of this muscle is at the border of the styloid process, and its fibers move forward, medially, and inferiorly to attach to the hyoid bone at the junction of the great horn of the bone (see Fig 1-52).

This muscle raises the hyoid bone and tongue. It also assists in depression of the mandible.

Head and cervical musculature

If the clinician is suspicious of some form of referred pain, or if the patient is complaining of some problem related to head posture, it is a good idea to palpate the muscles of the head[35] and neck, even though they are not directly implicated in masticatory function.

Empty-mouth movements

When examined individually, contacts between opposing teeth present a great deal of complexity. However, they may be basically evaluated as (1) centric positions and (2) eccentric positions. To promote understanding, it is useful to analyze the action of masticatory muscles during the sliding action of opposing teeth when there is no food in the mouth. On the other hand, functional activity during chewing may occur in centric or close-to-centric positions as well as when the mandible is approaching these centric positions. Figure 1-53 shows the spatial orientations of the masticatory muscles that are in charge of the activation of the mandible kinematics during empty movements of the jaw.

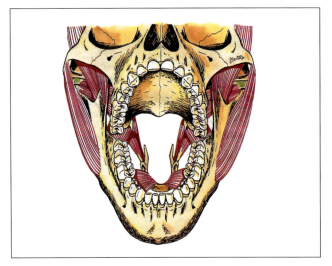

Fig 1-53 Masticator muscles in relation to cranial structures.

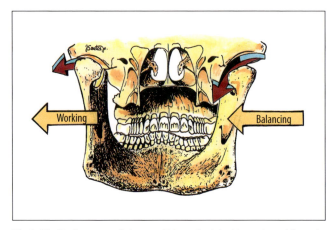

Fig 1-54 Displacement of the mandible to the left side as viewed from the back of the skull.

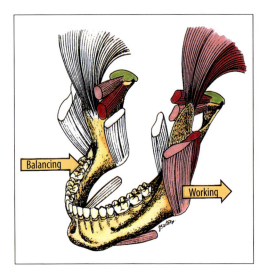

Fig 1-55 Action of masticatory muscles displacing the mandible to the left side. The vivid red represents the most potent contraction; the pink represents an assisting action of protagonist muscles. This color representation will be used consistently in the sequence of masticatory muscle action.

Lateral movement

If the jaw moves to the left side, this is considered the working side, and the condyle on the contralateral side (right side) would produce a balancing movement (Fig 1-54). Theoretically, the working condyle would be pivoting in its glenoid fossa, although some slight lateral displacement of the condyle can be produced.

For this movement to be produced, during a left lateral movement, the inferior head of the right lateral pterygoid muscle contracts and is assisted by the

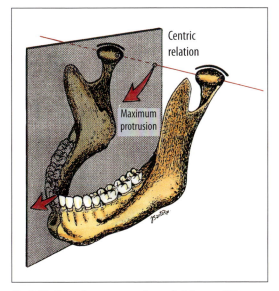

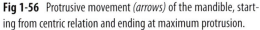

Fig 1-56 Protrusive movement *(arrows)* of the mandible, starting from centric relation and ending at maximum protrusion.

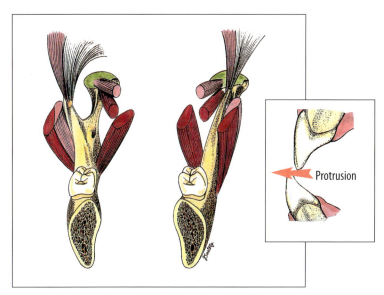

Fig 1-57 Action of masticatory muscles during protrusion of the mandible.

upper head of this same muscle. The upper head of the right lateral pterygoid is in charge of the anterior movement of the disc inside the joint as the right condyle moves forward in balancing translation. The inferior head of the right lateral pterygoid moves the right condyle forward. On the left side of the jaw, the deep layer of the masseter, the posterior bundle of the temporalis, and the superior head of the lateral pterygoid muscles are primarily activated to help to stabilize the condyle and corresponding disc inside the glenoid fossa. The superficial layer of the left masseter, the inferior head of the left lateral pterygoid, and the anterior belly of the digastric muscles assist in the production of smooth movement of the jaw during this displacement (Fig 1-55).

Protrusive movement

If a protrusive movement is imparted to the mandible, starting from centric position to maximum protrusion (Fig 1-56), there is bilateral activation of many masticatory muscles. During this movement, fibers of the superficial layer of the masseter, the medial pterygoid, and the inferior head of the lateral pterygoid muscles, on both sides of the head, are contracting simultaneously to project the jaw forward. This movement is assisted by the right and left superior heads of the lateral pterygoid muscles to produce synchronous forward movement of the discs in conjunction with translation of their respective condyles. The anterior bundles of both temporalis muscles also assist to control the smoothness of mandibular movement (Fig 1-57).

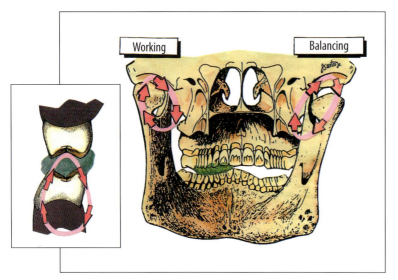

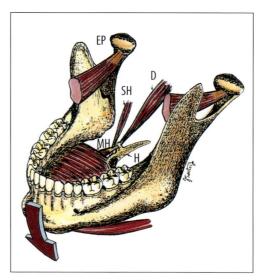

Fig 1-58 Example of left-side working chewing movement as viewed from the back of the skull. Note the movement of both working and balancing condyles, producing cyclic configurations *(arrows)*. *(inset)* The masticatory cycle has a teardrop shape at the level of the dentition.

Fig 1-59 Muscles in charge of mandibular depression *(arrow)*. (EP) External pterygoid muscle; (SH) stylohyoid muscle; (D) posterior belly of digastric muscle; (MH) mylohyoid muscle; (H) hyoid bone.

Retrusive movement

Voluntary mandibular retrusive movement can be achieved through bilateral contraction of the posterior bundles of the temporalis muscles and the deep layer of the masseters. If the movement starts from maximum protrusion, both lower heads of the lateral pterygoids are activated to help the mandibular retrusion. However, for this movement to be fully accomplished, the jaw must be braced in proper position through contraction of the suprahyoid musculature, and the hyoid bone must be stabilized.

Masticatory action

The masticatory cycle starts with the lowering of the mandible. At this mandibular position, with the exception of some selected muscles, the majority of the muscle fibers are at their optimal extent, producing the smallest volley of contractile impulses. From this point, selected muscles will be able to initiate elevation to reach tooth contact between opposing occlusal surfaces to accomplish crushing of the food. Apparently, at this stage, the muscles involved in the masticatory

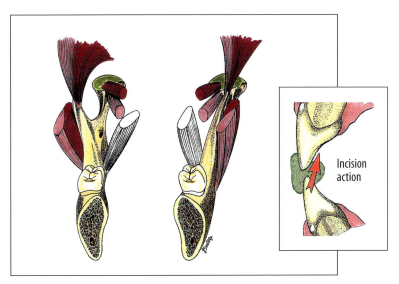

Fig 1-60 Action of masticatory muscles producing incision of the food.

action are starting their contraction, to achieve the maximal potential force and total intercuspation.

Movements during mastication are different from empty movements. For example, during a left-side masticatory cycle, the condylar movements involve circular paths for both balancing and working condyles (Fig 1-58). The balancing side translations are more extensive than the working side. These movements result in a teardrop-shaped configuration of the cyclic chewing movement produced at the dentition. The cyclic movement creates this teardrop shape when pantographic tracings are used. The apex of the teardrop is at the level of the opposing teeth during occlusion.

Incision of the food

When food is introduced to the mouth, the mandible is lowered because of the primary action of depressor muscles (Fig 1-59). The next step is the incision of the food. Bilateral, simultaneous, and synchronous contraction and relaxation of masticatory muscles occurs: contraction of the deep layer of the masseters, assisted by the superficial layers; contraction of the medial and posterior bundles of the temporalis, assisted by the anterior bundles; and contraction of the superior head of the lateral pterygoids, assisted by the inferior heads of the same muscles, which elevate and protract the mandible while opposing incisors are producing the incision (Fig 1-60).

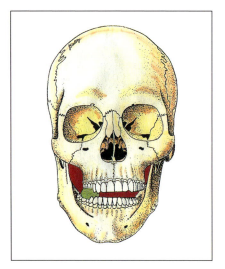

Fig 1-61 Right-side chewing.

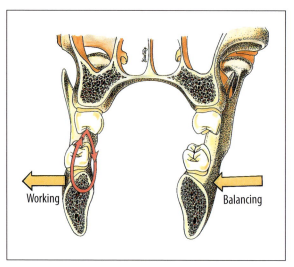

Working   Balancing

Fig 1-62 Right-side chewing.

Crushing of the food

With the first reduction of the food, the more specialized cycle of the mastication begins. The tongue and cheek muscles play an important role during mastication, to continuously position the food being crushed between occlusal surfaces.

If food is being chewed on the right side (Fig 1-61), for example, the mastication cycle continues with lowering and elevation of the mandible in a configuration similar to a teardrop (Fig 1-62). As mentioned before, the superior part of this teardrop is represented by the interocclusal contact between opposing teeth.

The masticatory cycle can be described in phases after the initial incision.

Phase 1: Opening

Phase 1 begins with the lowering, medial movement of the mandible. There is predominant bilateral contraction of the inferior head of the lateral pterygoid muscles, moving the condyles forward, assisted by the superior head of the lateral pterygoids, which in addition translate the discs forward in harmony with the condyles (Fig 1-63). The right lateral pterygoids and right medial pterygoid initially produce a more powerful contraction, moving the condyle forward and the mandible medially. Therefore, the main action of these muscles is to move the condyles forward. The accessory, suprahyoid musculature, especially the digastric muscles, are active in lowering the mandible. The masseter and temporalis muscles are practically inactive.

Fig 1-63 Phase 1. Lowering of the mandible *(arrow)*.

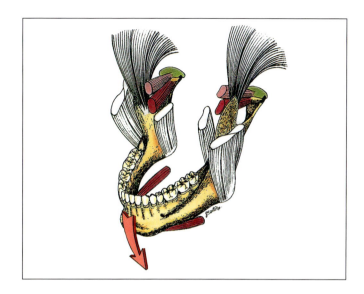

Fig 1-64 Phase 2. Closing phase of the mastication process. *(inset)* Lateral elevation of the mandible produces right-side chewing.

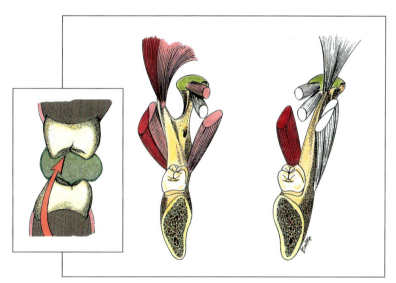

Phase 2: Closing

In phase 2, the mandible moves up and laterally to the right side. During this movement, muscles on both sides of the jaw are active. The left medial pterygoid is mobilized to help move the mandible to the right side. Simultaneously, on the right side, the superficial layer of the masseter and the anterior bundles of the temporalis (all assisted by the deep layer of the masseter, the intermediate and posterior bundles of the temporalis, the medial pterygoid, and the superior head of the lateral pterygoid muscles) promote mandibular elevation (Fig 1-64).

Phase 3: Occlusion

The occlusion phase of this cycle occurs with maximal masticatory muscle force on the right side of the mandible. At this stage, the forces generated by muscles are at their maximum potential. The occlusal tables of the teeth are deeply involved in this process. During this phase of mastication, the neuromuscular network is permanently active. This network consists of influential entities such as the periodontal membrane; TMJ capsule receptors; TMJ mechanoreceptors, the vascular supply, the limbic system, the brain stem, and the central nervous system, among other systems. These entities, acting as a whole, will provide the best control of events during the masticatory cycle, to deliver chewing continuity through an unconscious process. In the event of some problem, such as some threat to the peripheral structures of the masticatory system (for example, a piece of bone in the food), a reflex protective arch may be activated to interrupt the masticatory sequence.

During the occlusal masticatory phase, the strong action of the right-side muscles, including the superficial and deep layer of the masseters and the medial pterygoid (assisted by the temporalis muscle), promote grinding of the food. The working condyle in this event produces limited movements, while the action of the right superior head of the lateral pterygoid muscle (assisted by the right inferior head) generates rotation of the condyle and stabilization of the disc (Fig 1-65).

Although the description of this phase of the chewing cycle may seem to presume exclusively a group function relationship between posterior teeth, it seems clear that opposing occlusal surfaces come in contact during the masticatory act, with the involvement of cuspal inclines. However, if canine guidance is present, there is a predominance of axial masticatory loads at the depth of the opposing fossae, the result of which depends upon the long axis of the posterior teeth.

Phase 4: Exit

With the crushing stage of mastication concluded, the mandible moves down in the medial direction to clear away from the occlusal table of the opposing arch. Active action of the right medial pterygoid and both heads of the right lateral pterygoid muscles move the mandible medially. This movement, to control the speed of motion, is assisted by the superficial layer of the masseter and the anterior and intermediate bundles of the temporalis muscles, all on the right side of the mandible (Fig 1-66).

From this point on, a new cycle is started, beginning at phase 1. In general, in a healthy dentition, the subject has a tendency to shift sides for mastication, alternating between right and left chewing cycles.

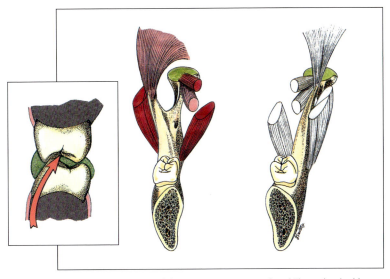

Fig 1-65 Phase 3. Occluding phase of the mastication process. *(inset)* The occlusal tables are deeply involved in crushing of the food.

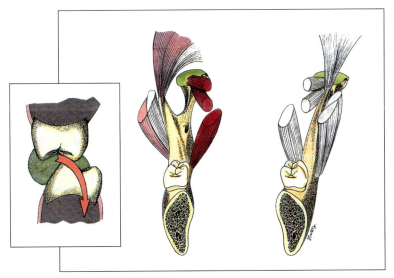

Fig 1-66 Phase 4. Exiting phase of mastication. *(inset)* The mandible starts to produce medial movement to allow the occlusal surfaces of opposing teeth to exit each other.

REFERENCES

1. Ash MM, Ramfjord SP. Occlusion, ed 4. Philadelphia: Saunders, 1995.
2. dos Santos J Jr. Occlusion: Principles and Concepts, ed 2. St Louis: Medico-Dental Media, 1998.
3. dos Santos J Jr. Temporomandibular disorders. In: Rakel RE (ed). Conn's Current Therapy 1998. Philadelphia: Saunders, 1998:986–990.
4. dos Santos J Jr. Occlusion: Principles and Concepts. St Louis: Ishiyaku EuroAmerica, 1985.
5. dos Santos J Jr. Oclusão Clínica Atlas Colorido [Clinical Occlusion Color Atlas]. São Paulo: Livraria Santos Editora, 1995.
6. Mohl ND, Zarb GA, Carlsson GE, Rugh JD. A Textbook of Occlusion. Chicago: Quintessence, 1988.
7. Nelson SJ, Nowlin TP (eds). Occlusion. Dent Clin North Am 1995;39(2):233–477.
8. Parker MW. Occlusal considerations in restorative dentistry. Curr Opin Dent 1991;1:192–198.
9. Rassouli NM, Christensen LV Experimental occlusal interferences. 3. Mandibular rotation induced by a rigid interference. J Oral Rehabil 1995;22:781–789.
10. Becker CM, Kaiser DA. Evolution of occlusion and occlusal instruments. J Prosthodont 1993;2:33–43.
11. Brecker SC. Clinical Procedures in Occlusal Rehabilitation, ed 2. Philadelphia: Saunders, 1966.
12. Dawson PE. Evaluation, Diagnosis, and Treatment of Occlusal Problems, ed 2. St Louis: Mosby, 1989.
13. Dickerson WG, Chan CA, Carlson J. The human stomatognathic system: A scientific approach to occlusion. Dent Today 2001;20(2):100–102,104–107.
14. dos Santos J Jr. Maxillofacial pains. In: Ash MM Jr (ed). Functional Occlusion II. Ann Arbor, MI: University of Michigan Dental Publications, 1987.
15. Gerber A, Steinhardt G. Dental Occlusion and the Temporomandibular Joint. Carmichael RP (trans). Chicago: Quintessence, 1990.
16. dos Santos J Jr. Seria a cárie dental o mal maior [webpage in Portuguese]? Available at: http://www.portugal-linha.pt/opiniao/Jsantos/cron1.html.
17. Lucia VO. Modern Gnathological Concepts, Updated. Chicago: Quintessence, 1983.
18. dos Santos J Jr, Blackman R, Nelson SJ. Vectorial analysis of the static equilibrium of forces generated in the mandible in centric occlusion, group function and balanced occlusion relationships. J Prosthet Dent 1991;65:557–567.
19. dos Santos J Jr, Silveira E. Stereophotogrammetry. Morphological study of the occlusal surface secondary grooves of posterior permanent teeth [in Portuguese]. Rev Fac Odontol São Paulo 1974;12:181–186.
20. dos Santos J Jr. Stereophotogrammetry. Study of the influence of mandibular movements in the volume of occlusal surface rehabilitation [in Portuguese]. 1. Rev Fac Odontol São Paulo 1975;13: 169–178.
21. dos Santos J Jr, Guidi D. Stereophotogrammetry. Study of the influence of mandibular movements in the volume of occlusal surface rehabilitation [in Portuguese]. 2. Rev Fac Odontol São Paulo 1976;14:35–40.
22. dos Santos J Jr, Matson E, Pancera AD. Stereometry. Study of mandibular movements in the determination of angular values of cuspal inclines [in Portuguese]. Rev Fac Odontol São Paulo 1977;15:45–52.
23. dos Santos J Jr, Fichman DM. Escultura e Modelagem Dental [Dental Carving and Modeling], ed 5. São Paulo: Livraria Santos Editora, 1989:chap 5.
24. dos Santos J Jr, de Rijk W. Occlusal contacts: Vectorial analysis of forces transmitted to temporomandibular joint and teeth. Cranio 1993;11:118–125.
25. Darlow LA, Pesco J, Greenberg MS. The relationship of posture to myofascial pain dysfunction syndrome. Am J Orthod Dentofac Orthop 1988;93:85–86.
26. American Academy of Prosthodontics. Glossary of Prosthodontic Terms. J Prosthet Dent 1994; 71:50–107.

27. Becker A, Karnei-R'em RM, Steigman S. The effects of infraocclusion. 3. Dental arch length and the midline. Am J Orthod Dentofacial Orthop 1992;102:427–433.

28. Arakawa Y, Yamaguchi H. Chewing movements in near ideal occlusion with and without TM symptoms. Cranio 1997;15:208–220.

29. Kuwahara T, Bessette RW, Maruyama T. Effect of continuous passive motion on the result of TMJ meniscectomy. 1. Comparison of chewing movement. Cranio 1996;14:190–199.

30. Lauret JF, Le Gall M. The function of mastication: A key determinant of dental occlusion. Pract Periodont Aesthet Dent 1996;8:807–818.

31. Goldberg LJ. Changes in the excitability of elevator and depressor motoneuron produced by stimulation of intra oral nerves. In: Anderson DJ, Mathews B (eds). Mastication. Bristol: Wright, 1976:165–173.

32. Abe S, Ouchi Y. Perspectives on the role of the lateral pterygoid muscle and the spheno-mandibular ligament in temporomandibular joint function. Cranio 1997;15:203–207.

33. Lafrenière CM, Lamontagne M, el Sawy R. The role of the lateral pterygoid muscles in TMJ disorders during static conditions. Cranio 1997;15:38–52.

34. Whatmore BG, Whatmore NJ, Fisher LD. Is frontalis activity a reliable indicator of the activity in other skeletal muscles? Biofeedback Self Regul 1981;6:305–314.

ARTICULATORS AND THEIR USES

Articulators are instruments (usually metal and sometimes with plastic components) capable of reproducing mandibular position and motions. They are tools the clinician uses for diagnosis and treatment of complex dental, jaw, and temporomandibular dysfunctional conditions. All articulators have different functions and mechanical restrictions. Different occlusal theories influence the designs, construction, and indications for use of different articulators. However, even considering the great variety of instruments available, it is likely that articulators may be consistent within the same category and constructed according to comparable standards.

Articulators are used to mount dental casts and simulate jaw movements. Procedures for mounting casts are analogous between instruments with minor differences, depending on the type of articulator. Structural variations are not germane when the clinician becomes familiar with the use of several different instruments.

The most important use of an articulator is for clinical dentistry. Before articulator use, it is indispensable to obtain occlusal records (intraoral or extraoral), hinge axis determinations, facebow transfer, and so on. If all records are accurate, the instrument will be able to simulate the movements of the patient's jaws dependably.

It is important that the mounted casts truly represent the conditions of the patient's mouth. The mounting must be correct. In the presence of certain disorders of the masticatory system, accurate recording of mandibular position is difficult. Correct mounting of casts in this case may be impossible. It is the clinician's challenge to evaluate and manage the patient to secure reproducible, accurate articulated casts. Therefore, the clinician is advised to provide symptomatic treatment for the patient (through the use of occlusal bite plane splints, for example)[1-7] or any other type of noninvasive treatment to alleviate the symptoms before mounting the casts or performing irreversible treatment procedures such as alteration of tooth structure.

There are two general classifications of articulators: *fully adjustable* and *semiadjustable* (including the simple axis instrument). There are two major types of semiadjustable articulator: arcon and non-arcon.

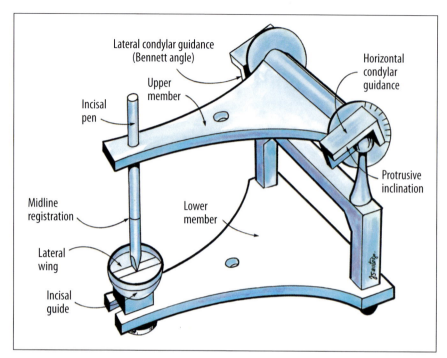

Fig 2-1 Hypothetical arcon semiadjustable articulator.

Arcon articulators reproduce the human anatomic maxillomandibular relationships of the skull; that is, the condylar balls of the instruments are coupled to each side of the vertical ramus of the lower frame. The articular elements (condylar housings) are located on each side of the upper frame of the instrument. In non-arcon articulators, the condylar balls are attached to the upper frame and the articular elements (condylar housings) are attached to the lower. Non-arcon articulators do not duplicate the anatomic features of the human skull.

The arcon articulator is the type most commonly used in dental practice. A hypothetical articulator, representing an arcon instrument, will be used in this chapter as an example (Fig 2-1).

All available semiadjustable articulators possess their own benefits and inconveniences. Their handling and effectiveness are distinguished by the expertise of the clinician. This chapter will describe the records needed for accurate transfer of the clinical situation to the articulator as well as the correct use and adjustment of the articulator.

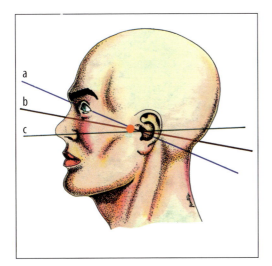

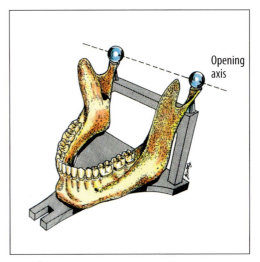

Fig 2-2 The *red dot* represents the lateral position of the horizontal arbitrary axis of rotation crossing both condyles. This axis also crosses the cranial reference planes. The cranial planes of reference are used for relating the maxillary cast to the upper member of the articulator. (a) Axio-canthus plane; (b) axio-orbital plane; (c) axio-ala plane.

Fig 2-3 Hinge opening of the jaw after being transferred to the articulator.

TRANSFER RECORDS

Hinge axis determination

A great number of instruments rely on an arbitrary hinge axis. For instance, the reference point for this arbitrary hinge axis may be measured 12 mm anterior from the tragus of the ear, on each side of the patient's head, and marked on a line that joins the external corner of the eye to the tragus. These points describe the approximate location of a virtual horizontal transverse axis of rotation through both condyles. This axis represents the fixed axis of mandibular rotation and is practically parallel to the frontal plane of the head (Fig 2-2). The three-dimensional location of this axis is transferred to the articulator (Fig 2-3).

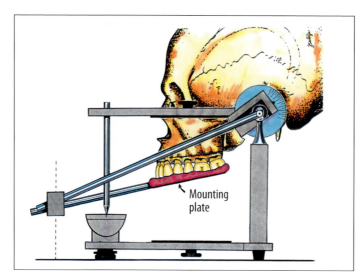

Fig 2-4 Relationship among the facebow, skull, and articulator.

Facebow records

Each articulator has a facebow.[8] This device is composed of several adjustable parts, which are mounted as a unit. The use of a facebow is very similar from articulator to articulator. The facebow is used to relate the maxillary arch, in a three-dimensional relationship, to the base of the skull (Fig 2-4). The facebow is positioned three-dimensionally by orienting it to three reference points on the face: two points on each side of the head and one anterior craniofacial point (Figs 2-2 and 2-5). These specific spatial relations enable the mounting of the maxillary cast to a definite, reproducible position in the articulator.

Essentially, a facebow is manufactured from a metal frame. Anterior to the middle distance of this frame, the stem of the mounting plate or clutch is braced; for some instruments, a transverse stylus is used as an indicator for the anterior cranial point of reference. The mounting plate is used to support the maxillary cast in position during its mounting on the upper member of the articulator. For better results during the facebow transfer, the stem of the mounting plate must be fixed at mid-distance within the anterior segment of the frame and positioned parallel to the sagittal plane of the patient.

The posterior lateral extremities of the frame, on each side of the head, may have styli that are related to the hinge axis position, marked beforehand at the level of the patient's temporomandibular joints (Fig 2-6). In some facebows the styli are replaced by earpieces, which are inserted in the external meatus of the ear.

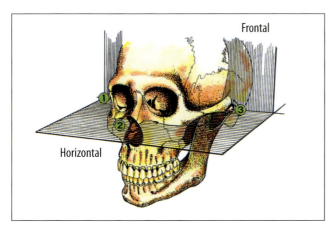

Fig 2-5 Intercondylar transverse axis (line 1-3) when the head is related to three-dimensional planes. (2) Third point of reference.

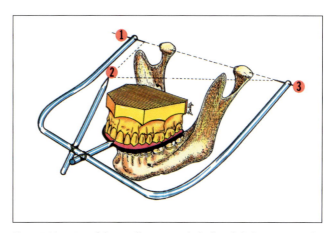

Fig 2-6 Mounting of the maxillary cast with the bite-fork. Points 1, 2, and 3 have the same relationships as represented in Fig 2-5.

Centric relation registration

Centric relation records guarantee the proper mounting of the mandibular cast in relation to the maxillary cast on the articulator. Although the interocclusal relations between maxillary and mandibular casts may be duplicated on the articulator by simply occluding the casts in maximum intercuspation (Fig 2-7), it is recommended that the casts be related with a centric relation record.[9,10] When accurately recorded, the centric relation interocclusal relationship will be a reproducible skeletal anatomic position between the maxilla and mandible. Furthermore, occlusal analysis, trial occlusal adjustment, complex rehabilitation procedures, and so on all involve the use of centric relation as an initial reference position for the clinical assessment of the dental occlusion and mandibular position.

The accurate determination of the centric relation position is relevant for several reasons. If casts are mounted on a fully adjustable or semiadjustable articulator, it is appropriate to secure a dependable centric relation location because it will provide a complete record of the interocclusal relationships. Centric relation, in some instances, will be the only way to transfer the interocclusal relationships to the articulator, predominantly when maximum intercuspation is not constant or even is not present. When comprehensive oral reconstruction is required, it is imperative to duplicate the maxillomandibular relationship for all plaster study cast mountings and remountings on the articulator to facilitate the process of diagnosis and treatment.

Manipulation of the mandible into centric relation is not always an easy procedure. Patients with certain conditions may not allow their masticatory muscles to

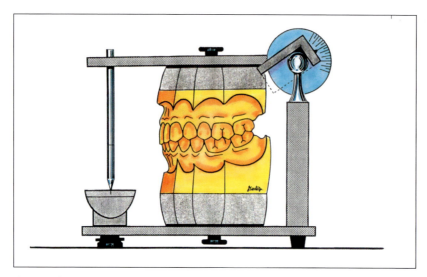

Fig 2-7 Relationship between maxillary and mandibular casts in intercuspal position. In this case, the mandibular cast was mounted on the articulator by simply occluding the casts in maximum intercuspation.

relax, and splinting action of the muscles will occur, producing relentless mandibular movements. Disorders of the masticatory system, a psychological reaction of the patient to any kind of manipulation of his or her mandible, poor patient cooperation, and other problems will make accurate centric relation registration very difficult. The patient must remain inactive during the gentle manipulation of the jaw into centric relation. Centric relation is not a forceful retruded position.

A good clinical method to increase the patient's level of relaxation is to ask the patient to occlude moderately on cotton rolls, on each side in the molar areas, for 10 to 15 minutes before any registration is undertaken. This approach may grant some brief "deprogramming" of the proprioceptive sensation of the mandible.

The process for registering centric relation starts with a relaxed seating position for the patient in the dental chair with the headrest adapted to the occipital area of the head. The backrest is inclined at a 45-degree angle in relation to the horizontal plane of the floor. For the best environment, it is beneficial to assure an atmosphere of relaxation for the patient, in which there is no needless noise or movement and the lighting is not too bright. With the use of a two-handed technique for mandibular manipulation, the clinician must secure a restful position behind the dental chair. The chin of the patient is accessed from behind, as the clinician uses each hand to hold one side of the mandible (Fig 2-8). Although experienced clinicians can use the one-handed technique, the two-handed technique is more dependable for directing the condyles into a consistent and reproducible transverse hinge axis, without the risk of deviation of the jaw to either side (Fig 2-9).

The clinician should practice with the patient before attempting to make a record. The lower border of the mandible is grasped with two hands. The patient is asked

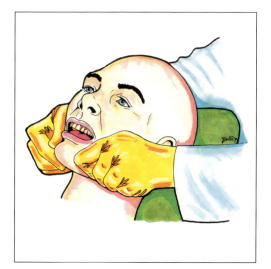

Fig 2-8 Two-handed technique for mandibular manipulation in centric relation.

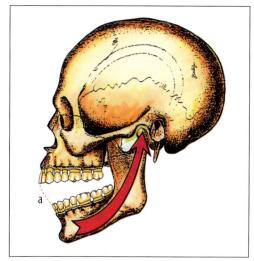

Fig 2-9 The proper manipulation of the mandible in centric relation along the opening arch (a) may cause distal displacement of the mandible, leading the condyles to a rearmost and uppermost position in the glenoid fossae *(arrow)*.

to slightly open the jaw and, with a mild and unstrained movement, the clinician directs the mandible backward and upward. Then, the clinician oscillates the mandible up and down with limited extension of jaw opening (no more than 2.5 mm at the level of opposing incisors). With slow motions, the clinician brings the mandible up to the first tooth contact in centric relation. If handling of the mandible is appropriate, there may be a slide from centric relation to maximum intercuspation (centric occlusion), especially if the patient is asked to contract his or her masticatory muscles during closure. Normally, this slide is no more extensive than 2.0 to 2.5 mm.

Centric relation occlusal record

The following procedure is used to make an intraoral occlusal record of the centric relation position. There are also extraoral techniques for this registration that will not be discussed here.

The substance (usually wax) used for registration must not distort the maxillomandibular relationship during recording. Dead-soft baseplate wax, uniformly softened at 138°F in a water bath, is used.

While the patient's mouth is open, a piece of gauze is used to dry the occlusal surfaces of the maxillary teeth. The softened wax waffle is now cautiously adapted to the occlusal surfaces of the maxillary teeth. Molding the buccal overhang of the wax into the buccal and labial embrasures will secure the waffle. In partially edentulous patients, additional wax is added to the edentulous areas for support of the wax waffle.

Without delay, before cooling of the wax, the mandible is manipulated into centric relation to create the indentations. Most if not all of the teeth should be recorded so that good seating of casts will be feasible.

Avoid any show-through of the wax, because opposing teeth should not contact during the recording. However, in most cases, the thickness of the waffle used for recording must not exceed 3 mm (or three layers of baseplate wax). Soft tissue encroachment must be avoided during recording.

The horseshoe-shaped configuration for the wax record (Fig 2-10) is preferable because it avoids encroachment on the soft tissues in the lingual portion of the casts. After the teeth are imprinted in the warm wax, the registration material should be set aside to firm at room temperature to prevent warping during handling and mounting procedures. After being chilled and trimmed, the registration must be rechecked in the mouth.

Mandibular protrusion registration

For the proper use of articulators, it is necessary to record protrusive mandibular displacement. The settings of condylar inclination are adjusted with protrusive recordings. Most articulators use this type of recording for this adjustment.

The use of an intraoral wax record of mandibular protrusion is very simple and is made by the same precepts described in the previous section. Some patients have an anatomic configuration of the jaws that provides great clearance between opposing posterior teeth when the mandible is protruded. In such cases, sufficient layers of wax must be added to the wax rim so that regular and positive indentations can be registered.

Reproducible protrusive movements are recorded when dental casts are related and mounted according to the hinge axis of the articulator (and the centric relation of the patient). As a starting point, the clinician should allow the patient to practice performing reproducible protrusive movements. It is critical to examine the amount of deviation of the mandible to either side of the head. The midline between maxillary and mandibular central incisors can be used as reference. The protrusive registration must conform to centric relation alignment. Any deviation may be marked with a felt-tipped pen on the maxillary incisor. A hand mirror is useful in helping the patient to guide the mandible in protrusion according to this alignment (Fig 2-11).

The extension of the mandible in protrusion must never go any further than the edge-to-edge position (unless the patient has a Class III malocclusion). Any extension of movement beyond this limit will result in an erroneous record because the condylar housings on articulators restrict movement of the condyles.

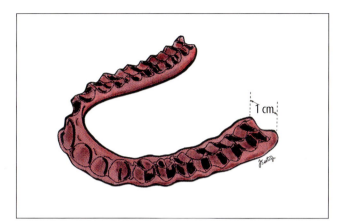

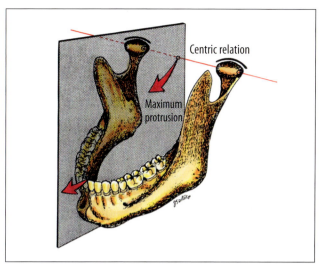

Fig 2-10 Typical appearance of a centric wax bite registration used to mount the casts on the articulator. When made with three layers of wax, this registration will provide a 1- to 2-mm clearance between the maxillary and mandibular casts.

Fig 2-11 Proper alignment of the mandible for the protrusive record, where both condyles move forward *(arrows)* to maximum protrusion evenly from centric relation. The protrusive registration must coincide with centric relation, even in midline deviation cases, from maximum intercuspation.

Lateral records (checkbites)

Most articulators have provision for a Bennett angle setting. To adjust the respective condylar elements for the Bennett angle, some instruments require lateral records in both right and left lateral movements.

Procedures during registration are comparable to those explained in the previous sections. The limit of mandibular displacement to either side is governed by the alignment of labial cusps of opposing canines (in canine-guided occlusion) and buccal cusps of posterior teeth (in group function).

ARTICULATOR TECHNIQUE

Baseline settings

The articulator should be checked before each use for its baseline setting, sometimes called *zeroing* the instrument. However, *zeroing* is not the most precise word to describe this maneuver, because not all elements of the instruments are set in

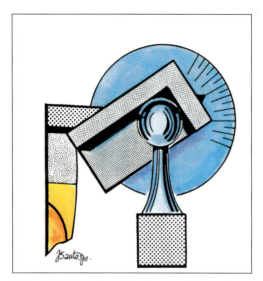

Fig 2-12 Articular and condylar elements of the articulator.

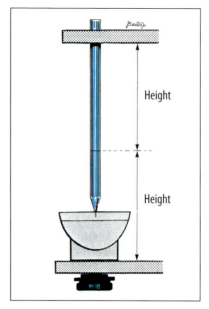

Fig 2-13 Incisal pin and incisal table assembly. The height of the upper and lower members of the instrument should be equal.

the zero position before casts are mounted. Rather, some movable parts of the instrument are centered or adjusted to preliminary (or baseline) settings.

Dental casts are often mounted and remounted several times during complex restorative dentistry. Hence, any restorative process completed using an articulator that was not properly adjusted according to its baseline settings will probably be imprecise.

The following is a series of steps to provide the baseline setting of the instrument:

1. Each condylar ball should be centered in its condylar housing and resting against its condylar stop (Fig 2-12). This represents the first requirement for articulator preparation.
2. In Fig 2-12, the horizontal condylar guidance is set at a certain angle (probably 30 degrees). The angle in this case is not consequential, but most articulator manufacturers recommend setting the horizontal condylar guidance at an angle greater than 0 degrees.
3. With lateral condylar guidance set at 0 degrees, the incisal pin should be seated on the center of the incisal table as a visual and functional reference (Fig 2-13).
4. It is also necessary to have the incisal pin centered at an anterior-posterior position on the incisal table (see Fig 2-13). If is not centered, the incisal table should be loosened and moved back and forth until the central position is achieved.

5. The height of the incisal pin must be adjusted to maintain the upper and lower members (or frames) of the articulator parallel between each other. Most incisal pins have a surrounding mark or notch to aid in the accomplishment of this task.
6. The incisal table must be in the horizontal position and the respective wings should be set at 0 degrees.

Mounting the casts

Maxillary cast

Once the articulator is prepared and the condylar elements are stabilized, the instrument is placed in a stable position on the bench and the upper frame is opened. The facebow is connected to the instrument. The top of the maxillary cast is scored with a sharp instrument and soaked in water for a few minutes. The maxillary cast is secured to the indentations on the wax used for bite registration (or low-fusing compound) and adapted to the mounting plate or clutch. Quick-setting mounting plaster is applied to the top of the cast and retentive areas of the mounting ring. It is important to use an amount of plaster just sufficient to secure the maxillary cast in position. Next, the upper member of the articulator is closed onto the cast on the facebow bite fork. The incisal pin is made to contact the incisal table (or the upper member is made to contact the facebow, depending on the type of articulator) (see Fig 2-4).

Once the plaster is completely set, the facebow is detached. Excess plaster should be trimmed from the cast. If required, extra plaster may be added to anchor the cast firmly in position.

Mandibular cast

After the maxillary cast is mounted on the articulator, the facebow is no longer needed. The next step is to mount the mandibular cast on the lower frame of the instrument. The condylar balls must rest against the condylar stops.

The upper and lower frames of the articulator should be parallel. As mentioned earlier, some instruments have notches (reference marks) on the incisal pin, to guide the operator to define this parallelism. When the mandibular cast is ready to be mounted (with the intraoral centric relation wax record), the incisal pin must be elongated by 3 to 5 mm to compensate for the thickness of the wax bite record (if the pin has the reference mark, this elongation will be above the reference).

For this procedure, the instrument is placed upside down and the frames are opened. The centric relation registration is adapted to the maxillary cast. The base of the mandibular cast is scored and soaked in water. In sequence, adjust

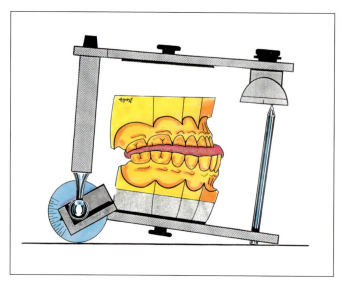

Fig 2-14 Mounting of the mandibular cast using a centric relation bite registration.

the mandibular cast to the indentations of the wax registration (Fig 2-14). While the cast is held firmly against the indentations, the stability of the cast against the bite recording should be checked. As an extra precaution, the mandibular cast can be braced against the indentations with rubber bands, strings, impression plaster, sticky wax, wooden sticks, or any other material that can be easily removed later. Quick-setting mounting plaster is applied to the base of the mandibular cast and in the retentive grooves of the mounting ring. Additional plaster is applied to the base of the cast. The articulator is closed; the incisal pin must be contacting the incisal table.

Verifying the precision of the mounting

It is important to remember that the precision of the mounting may be checked only after the horizontal condylar guidance is set. At the conclusion of the mounting, both casts will be fixed in centric relation. To verify the precision of the mounting, the articulator is adjusted so that the casts are in the intercuspal position. Next, the incisal pin is set at the level of the vertical dimension of occlusion (Fig 2-15). At this stage, the articulator is adjusted to the correct vertical dimension.

To assure the correct intercuspal position of the casts, the thumbnut screw holding the upper ring is loosened while the members of the articulator are held together. If the casts have a tendency to wobble, the centric relation record was not accurate, or the patient does not have a stable intercuspal position.

If the mandibular cast is mounted in centric relation (for the patient with a slide in centric), then the condylar balls of the articulator will not contact the condylar

Fig 2-15 Examination of the maximum inter-cuspation contacts after mounting of the mandibular cast. *(inset)* Note the anterior displacement of the condylar sphere (element) when the casts are in intercuspal position.

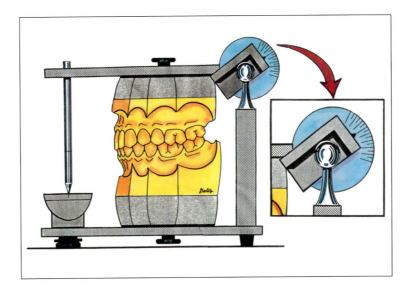

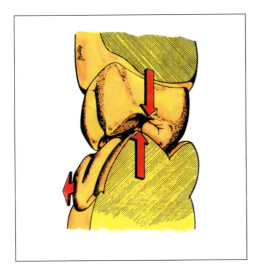

Fig 2-16 Centric relation contact relationship. This relationship must be accurately reproduced in the articulator. *Vertical arrows* show orientation of supporting cusps in centric relation; *horizontal arrow* shows tendency for distal displacement of mandibular cast in centric relation.

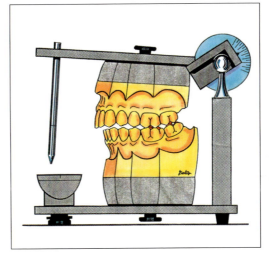

Fig 2-17 When the casts are placed in centric relation position, producing the first contact in centric relation, the incisal pin does not touch the incisal table.

stops when opposing casts are placed in the intercuspal position. However, the incisal pin will contact the incisal table, provided that the table is flat and without any inclination (see Fig 2-15). If the articulator is now guided into centric relation position, the occlusal surfaces of the posterior teeth will be in an unstable position (Figs 2-16 and 2-17). At this moment, the incisal pin moves forward and upward and is no longer contacting the incisal table (see Fig 2-17). The incisal pin assumes this

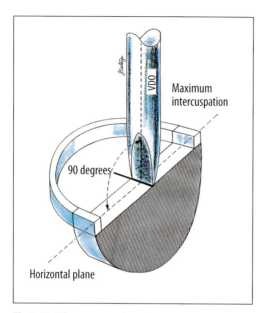

Fig 2-18 When casts are in maximum intercuspation, it is necessary to adjust the vertical dimension of occlusion (VDO). This is achieved by extending the incisal pin to touch the center of the incisal table.

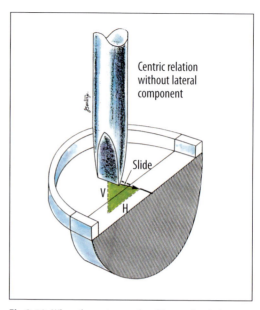

Fig 2-19 When the casts are related in centric relation contact, the incisal pin does not touch its respective incisal table. If there is no lateral deviation from centric relation to maximum intercuspation, it is possible to observe only the horizontal (H) and vertical (V) components of the slide.

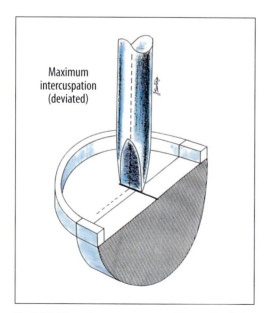

Fig 2-20 When the casts are mounted in centric relation and there is a midline deviation in maximum intercuspation, this can be detected at the level of the incisal pin and incisal table. The pin will be skewed to one side of the center of the incisal table.

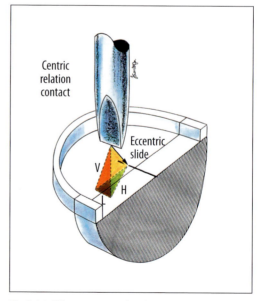

Fig 2-21 When casts are related to first contact in centric relation, the pin does not touch the incisal table but will assume a centered position in relation to its respective table. In this case, it is possible to observe that the eccentric slide displays a lateral component (L). (H) horizontal; (V) vertical.

spatial relationship because of the slide in centric (Figs 2-18 and 2-19). Variations of the occlusal slide can be detected at the level of the incisal table, when the incisal pin is calibrated to the appropriate vertical dimension of occlusion and the mandible deviates to one of the sides (Figs 2-20 and 2-21).

Another method of verifying the precision of the mounting is to use articulating ribbon to inspect the number of centric stops when the casts are gently tapped in the intercuspal position and compare the results to those found in the patient's occlusion. During impression procedures, the teeth sustain a position in their alveolar cavities that is different from their position when the patient occludes. As a result, more centric stops will be recorded in the mouth than on the casts.

Adjustments

Horizontal condylar guidance for protrusive movements

The next procedure uses the protrusive record to set the angulations of the horizontal condylar guidance (Fig 2-22). The horizontal condylar guidance of the articulator can be slanted to simulate the path of the condyle and articular disc in the glenoid fossa. This anterior inclination of the articulator is measured in degrees and exemplifies a relative measurement, rather than an absolute value. That is, articulated dental casts are a mechanical counterpart of jaw movements and may be apt to simulate functional actions of the mandible to a certain degree. Therefore, when casts are mounted on an articulator, they assume the same spatial relationship as the teeth have to the base of the skull. Likewise, the anterior inclination of the articulator should simulate the anterior inclination of the articular eminence (Fig 2-23). To adjust the guidance, when the protrusive record is stabilized between casts, first the left and then the right horizontal condylar guidance is rotated up and down. Then, each one is brought into contact with its respective condylar spheres. This procedure is controlled with both tactile and visual inspection. There will be only one setting at which the casts will be stabilized on the protrusive record (Fig 2-24).

The horizontal condylar guidance, which has an individual reading for each side of the head (but within small differences), maintains proportions in relation to the plane of occlusion (see Fig 2-23). In most patients, the slope of the angle of the horizontal condylar guidance is steep compared to the inclination of the plane of occlusion.

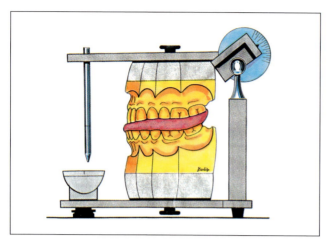

Fig 2-22 Use of the protrusive wax bite registration to adjust the horizontal condylar guidance inclination.

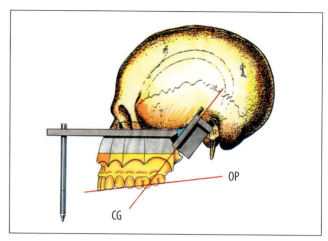

Fig 2-23 Relationship of the articular element of the upper member and the mounted cast superimposed on the skull. The red lines represent the condylar guidance (CG) and occlusal plane (OP) as related to the anatomic structures of the temporomandibular joint and articular element of the articulator. The anterior inclination of the eminence is supposed to be similar to that of the articulator to reproduce mandibular motions.

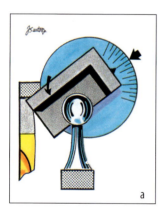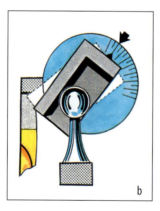

Fig 2-24 Use of the protrusive wax bite registration to adjust the horizontal condylar guidance. *Short arrows* indicate changes in angulation of condylar guidance. *(a)* A downward rotation *(curved arrow)* of the articular element (condylar housing) is started to make the lower surface of the guidance touch the sphere of the articulator, with the wax bite registration in position. *(b)* Forced downward rotation of the articular element should be avoided, because this procedure may dislodge the posterior portion of the casts. The final adjustment is achieved when there is no "rocking" between casts.

Lateral condylar guidance for the Bennett angle

Another mechanical counterpart of anatomic conditions offered by adjustable articulators is the ability to adjust the lateral condylar guidance for the Bennett angle. The lateral guidance can be calculated with the Hanau formula:

$$\text{Lateral condylar guidance} = \frac{\text{Horizontal condylar guidance}}{8} + 12$$

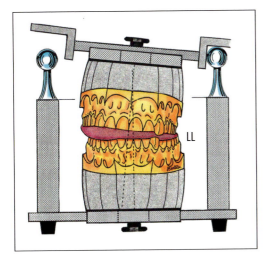

Fig 2-25 Use of a left lateral checkbite (LL) to adjust the right-side Bennett angle of the condylar housing.

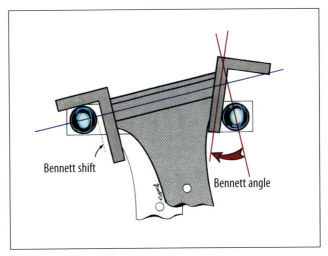

Fig 2-26 View of the articulator from above. A right lateral checkbite in this example was used to set the left Bennett angle of the condylar housing. Note the space formed between the condylar sphere and the condylar housing on the right side of the instrument. This movement, the Bennett shift, is a typical mechanical equivalent of lateral jaw displacement, which may be reproduced by the majority of the articulators during eccentric movements.

To set the left and right lateral condylar guidances of the articulator, the condylar housing is loosened and then each one is adjusted to its corresponding calculated value. However, if lateral checkbites for right and left displacements of the mandible are used (Fig 2-25), the lateral wall of each corresponding side's condylar housing should touch the condylar sphere (Fig 2-26).

Differences in the Bennett angle, when the angle of the condylar guidance is constant, may strongly influence the occlusal relationships between casts in working and balancing movements. These differences may also influence the amount of the side shift with reference to the transverse axis of the articulator. For example, if the Bennett angle is low, at 5 degrees (Fig 2-27), during the left working displacement of the articulator (Fig 2-28), there will be an almost straight lateral movement of the tip of the supporting cusp of the mandibular molar as it moves away from the central fossa of the maxillary molar. The side shift displacement of the working condyle is minimal. If the articulator is moved to the left balancing movement (Fig 2-29), the tip of the supporting cusp of the mandibular molar will move forward and will not compromise the supporting cusp of the maxillary molar. There is little tendency for balancing contact in this case.

In another example, if the Bennett angle is increased to 25 degrees (Fig 2-30), during left working movement of the articulator (Fig 2-31), the tip of the supporting

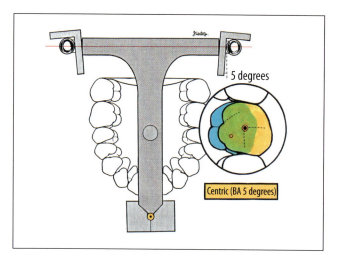

Fig 2-27 View of the articulator from above, showing the relationship of the upper member to the lower member in maximum intercuspation (centric occlusion). In this drawing and Figs 2-28 to 2-32, note the details of the articular elements and the outline of the occlusal surfaces, which are shown in yellow and blue (superimposition in green). Cusp tips are represented by *black dots* and centric stops by *red circles*. The Bennett angle (BA) in this case is set at 5 degrees.

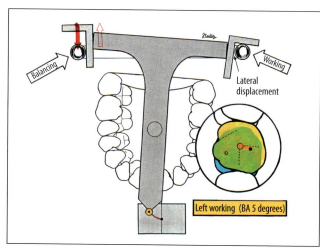

Fig 2-28 The articulator setup is the same as that shown in Fig 2-27, but the upper frame has been moved to a position of left working movement. The Bennett angle (BA) is set at 5 degrees. *Red arrows* indicate back and forth displacement of the right condylar sphere on the balancing side of the articulator during left working movement.

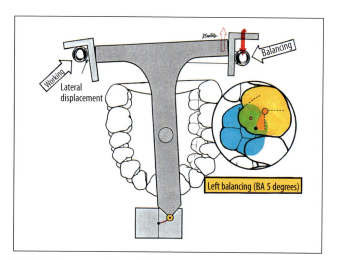

Fig 2-29 The same articulator has been moved to a left balancing position. The Bennett angle (BA) is set at 5 degrees. *Red arrows* indicate back and forth movement of the condylar sphere on the left balancing side of the articulator during right working movement.

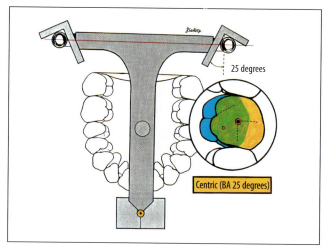

Fig 2-30 The articulator is in maximum intercuspation (centric occlusion), but the Bennett angle (BA) is set at 25 degrees.

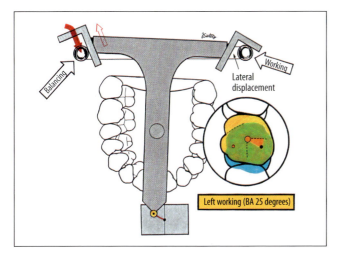

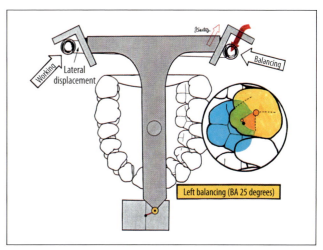

Fig 2-31 The articulator has been moved to left working movement. The Bennett angle (BA) is set at 25 degrees. *Red arrows* represent the back and forth displacement of the right condylar sphere on the balancing side of the articulator during right working movement.

Fig 2-32 The articulator has been moved to left balancing position. The Bennett angle (BA) is set at 25 degrees. *Red arrows* represent back and forth displacement of the right condylar sphere on the balancing side of the articulator during left working movement.

cusp of the mandibular molar will produce a more encompassing lateral movement with an increased tendency for balancing-side interference. The amount of side shift at the level of the working condyle will increase considerably. If there is a movement to left balancing side (Fig 2-32), there will be a sweeping movement of the tip of the supporting cusp of the mandibular molar to contact the opposing cusp tip of the maxillary molar. In this case, there is a great tendency for balancing contact.

The incidence of balancing contact will depend on the compensatory setting of the condylar guidance angle. The greater the angle of the condylar guidance, the greater will be the Bennett angle. Consequently, an increase of the Bennett angle will increase the incidence of balancing contacts and side shift. These differences may have a profound influence on the determination and adjustment of occlusal patterns during oral rehabilitation procedures.

Fischer angle

The three dimensions of the Fischer angle are oriented to the facial sagittal plane. However, there is no way to adjust the articular elements of the majority of articulators according to this angle. Most articulators are only oriented to the two-dimensional anterior-posterior movement of the condyles and the corresponding Bennett angles.

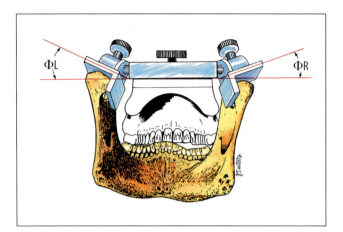

Fig 2-33 Posterior view of the Fischer angle settings, left (ΦL) and right (ΦR), on a hypothetical articulator. The condylar guidance of the upper member is adjusted according to the left working mandibular movement, determining the corresponding angles.

A few articulators have a provision to allow setting of the Fischer angle. The instruments that enable this adjustment permit the rotation of their corresponding articular elements laterally, downward, and medially to contact their respective condylar spheres, representing the mandibular condyles (Fig 2-33).

Intercondylar distance

There are numerous concerns about the influence of the intercondylar distance during oral rehabilitations. The most common question is if it is essential to ensure the accurate intercondylar distance when semiadjustable articulators are utilized. Some facebows (for example, the Whip-Mix facebow) are marked to specify the intercondylar distance as small, medium, or large. A question arises when the measurement does not correspond exactly to the interval on the facebow: Should the large or small distance be selected?

When circumstances prescribe the use of semiadjustable articulators, experience indicates that the choice of intercondylar distance may introduce possible changes on the occlusal surfaces of teeth being restored. The shorter the intercondylar distance, the greater the likelihood for occlusal grooves and inclines to be dislodged distally on maxillary teeth and mesially on mandibular teeth.[9] These outcomes may bias the definitive adjustment of occlusal configurations on the nonworking side when the patient has a very precise relationship in this position. Consequently, it is prudent to avoid the use of a smaller intercondylar distance when faced with a decision.

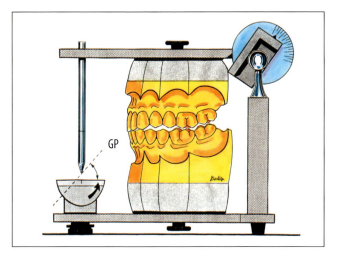

Fig 2-34 When the incisal guide pin (GP) and incisal table are adjusted for protrusive movement *(arrow)*, the articulator must be moved according to the anterior tooth guidance during this movement.

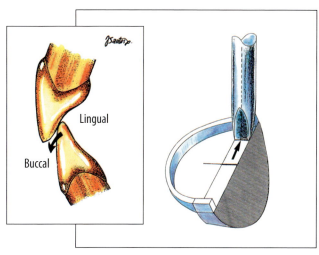

Fig 2-35 Adjustment of the incisal pin and incisal table in protrusive movement. *(inset)* The anterior tooth guidance aids in the adjustment.

Incisal guidance

The incisal pin and incisal table of the articulators are also mechanical counterparts that are adjustable. The incisal table of articulators can be inclined and adjusted to guide the incisal pin. In general, the incisal table can be adjusted to a positive inclination of 60 degrees and a negative inclination of 20 degrees. This adjustment is set when the casts are moved into protrusive and lateral positions. It is imperative to adjust the protrusive guidance first (adjust the tilting of the table) and then to adjust the guidance for lateral movements (adjust the elevation of the wings). The incisal guidance is set to simulate tooth guidance when tooth structures are not present or to preclude wear of the casts during manipulation of the articulator. The incisal pin never clears the table during eccentric movements.

The restriction imposed by the incisal table may eventually require the clinician to customize the incisal guidance with quick-cured acrylic resin or visible light–cured resin composites (used to fabricate trays). Incisal guidance trajectories are grooved in the softened material with the round tip of the incisal pin during functional sliding movements of the casts. The customized, incisal guidance is obtained when the material hardens.

Protrusive movements
The anterior inclination of the incisal table is set when casts are protruded (Fig 2-34). The maxillary and mandibular incisors are used for anterior guidance. The articulator must produce a gliding movement between the lingual surfaces and incisal edges of opposing incisors (Fig 2-35).

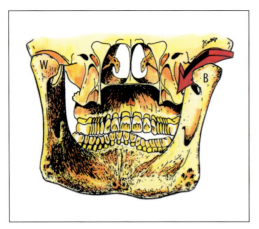

Fig 2-36 Posterior view of the skull, showing the balancing (B) and working (W) relationships of the condyles. *Arrow* indicates medial displacement of the condyle during balancing movement.

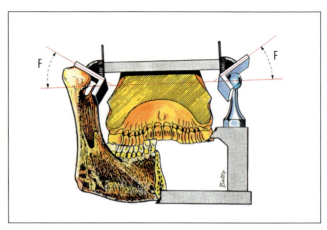

Fig 2-37 Posterior view of the skull in combination with the articulator. Note the spatial relationship of the condylar housing when adjusted to the mechanical equivalent of condylar motion. Other angular values may be measured in this case, such as the Fisher angle (F).

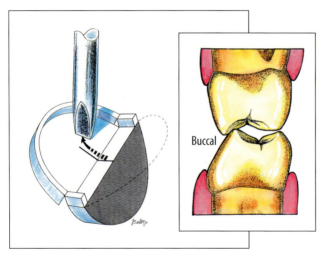

Fig 2-38 Frontal view of the lateral movement *(arrow)* between casts guided by the incisal pin and incisal table. *(inset)* The molar relationship may influence the adjustment of the lateral wings of the incisal table. The incisal pin and incisal table adjustment in this example provide guidance for right working movement when the patient has group function.

Lateral movements

Right and left eccentric movements of the mandible (Fig 2-36) are related to the condylar guidance of the articulator. The setting of the condylar housing of the articulator may also produce three-dimensional relationships that may reveal different angular readings, such as, for example, the Fisher angle (Fig 2-37). These settings are supposed to correspond to the existing interocclusal relationships of the patient and allow proper contact of the incisal pin against the wings of the incisal table (Fig 2-38).

REFERENCES

1. Boero RP. The physiology of splint therapy: A literature review. Angle Orthod 1990;59:165–180.
2. Carossa S, Di Bari E, Lombardi M, Preti G. A graphic evaluation of the intermaxillary relationship before and after therapy with the Michigan splint. J Prosthet Dent 1990;63:586–592.
3. dos Santos J Jr, Suzuki H, Ash MM Jr. Mechanical analysis of the equilibrium of occlusal splints. J Prosthet Dent 1988;59:346–352.
4. Guinn JL, Williams BT. Choosing the right appliance. J Craniomandib Pract 1985;3:289–293.
5. McCarroll RS, Naeije M, Kim YK, Hansson TL. The immediate effect of splint-induced changes in jaw positioning on the asymmetry of submaximal masticatory muscle activity. J Oral Rehabil 1989;16:163–170.
6. McCarroll RS, Naeije M, Kim YK, Hansson TL. Short-term effect of a stabilization splint on the asymmetry of submaximal masticatory muscle activity. J Oral Rehabil 1989;16:171–176.
7. Tsuga K, Akagawa Y, Sakaguchi R, Tsuru H. A short-term evaluation of the effectiveness of stabilization-type occlusal splint therapy for specific symptoms of temporomandibular joint dysfunction syndrome. J Prosthet Dent 1989;61:610–613.
8. dos Santos J Jr, Nelson S, Nummikoski P. Geometric analysis of occlusal plane orientation using simulated ear-rod facebow transfer. J Prosthodont 1996;5:172–181.
9. dos Santos J Jr, Nelson S, Nowlin T. Comparison of condylar guidance setting obtained from wax record and extraoral tracing. A pilot study. J Prosthet Dent 2003;89:54–60.
10. dos Santos J Jr, de Rijk W. Vectorial analysis of the instantaneous equilibrium of forces between incisal and condylar guidances. Cranio 1992;10:305–312.

DIFFERENTIAL DIAGNOSIS OF MAXILLOFACIAL PAIN

Irrespective of the location in the body, pain may be a significant part of human suffering. Unlike other normal physiologic senses (smell, taste, touch, vision, and hearing), it represents a state of neurologic distress, which can result from local trauma; inflammatory processes; accumulation of toxic substances in the tissues (eg, bradykinin, lactic acid, histamine, potassium ions); ischemia; mechanical deformation; and other causes.

There are a variety of pain experiences that may involve the maxillofacial structures. These types of pain are of special significance to the dental profession not only because of the area of the body affected but also because of their complexity and misleading presentations, which may represent a significant challenge to the clinician who is attempting to determine the cause of the problem.[1–22]

MAXILLOFACIAL NEURAL PATHWAYS

Impulses arising from the peripheral structures are carried to the central nervous system through afferent fibers of large and small diameter (Figs 3-1 and 3-2). In general, large-diameter myelinated fibers (mechanoreceptor and touch conductors) have their impulses filtered in the ipsilateral spinal nucleus of the fifth (trigeminal) nerve after traversing the spinal tract of this same nerve, where the gate control mechanism is believed to be located (Figs 3-3 and 3-4). For more complete information about theories of pain mechanism, the reader is encouraged to refer to detailed textbooks on the subject.[2,3,16,17,23–25]

Superficially on the face and head, there are precise boundaries of regions innervated by ophthalmic, maxillofacial, and mandibular branches of the sensory portion of the trigeminal nerve. In addition, these boundaries contain tissues overlying the posterior-lateral and inferior portions of the mandible that are innervated by the dorsal root of the second and third cervical nerves. This complex system of innervation creates a laminated arrangement of craniofacial dermatomes (Fig 3-5).

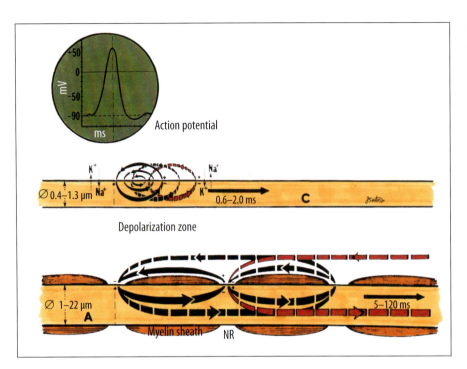

Fig 3-1 Small- and large-diameter fibers, where a stimulus is applied, depolarizing the nerve membranes, thus producing an impulse or action potential that spreads along the membranes in a wavelike fashion. The large-diameter myelinated fibers (A) have greater conductance than the small ones (C), because of the saltatory conduction effect during the propagation of the impulses through the nodes of Ranvier (NR).

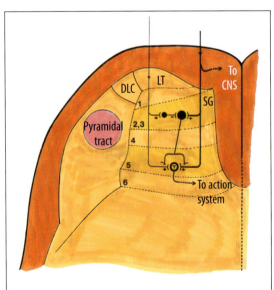

Fig 3-2 Synaptic gate in the dorsal column. The substantia gelatinosa (SG) is located in lamina 2 and 3 and represents part of the active portion of the gate control mechanism. In lamina 5, the transmission cells (T) are located. (CNS) Central nervous system; (LT) Lissauer tract; (DLC) dorsal lateral column.

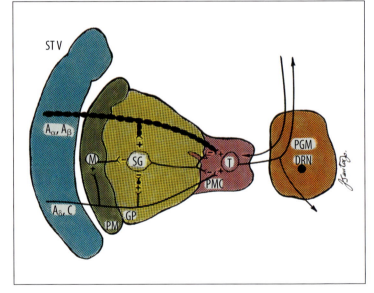

Fig 3-3 Trigeminal nerve (V) sensory pathways according to the gate control theory. (ST V) Spinothalamic tract of the trigeminal nerve; (A_α, A_β) large-diameter myelinated nerve fiber; (A_δ, C) small-diameter nonmyelinated nerve fiber; (M) modulating interneuron; (PM) pars marginalis or first lamina; (GP) gelatinous parts or second and third laminae; (PMC) pars magnocellularis or fifth lamina; (SG) substantia gelatinosa rolandi; (T) transmission cell; (PGM) periaqueductal gray matter; (DRN) dorsal raphe nucleus.

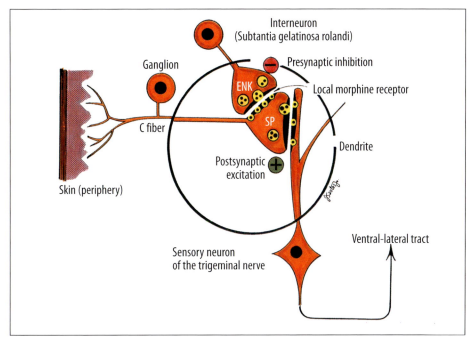

Fig 3-4 Peripheral sensorial transmission of nerve impulses to the central nervous system through a synaptic transmission of the dendrites of the fifth nerve. It represents the release of substance P (SP) at the level of the excitatory postsynaptic junction. Note the modulator presynaptic inhibition of an interneuron in the substantia gelatinosa rolandi, releasing enkephalin (ENK).

Fig 3-5 Laminated arrangement of the facial innervations (dermatome). (Ophth) Ophthalmic branch of the trigeminal nerve; (Max) maxillary branch of the trigeminal nerve; (Mand) mandibular branch of the trigeminal nerve; (Cerv) branches 2, 3, 4, and 5 of the cervical nerve.

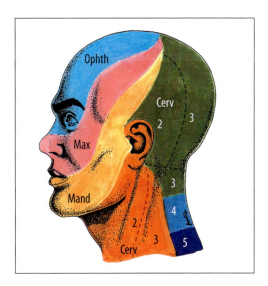

Referred pain mechanism

As a general rule, acute pain may be felt at the primary site of noxious stimulation. In some instances, pain may be felt in an anatomic area detached from the primary area of injury. This phenomenon is called *referred pain* and may occur at a point distant from the site of the damage. It also occurs through summation mechanisms influencing other neural segments. However, the theory of excitation to the central nervous system provides the best basis for the explanation of this type of pain.

According to the theory of excitation, a barrage of painful sensory impulses reaching the central nervous system may excite nearby and dormant internuncial neurons, producing a reaction.

The clinical incidence of this effect appears to occur almost exclusively when the main source of pain arises in areas other than peripheral structures.[1,2,3,8]

Spreading pain mechanism

There are some studies suggesting that a *convergence pattern* (Fig 3-6) mechanism may underlie the spread of pain that is frequently observed in pain conditions affecting the orofacial structures and headaches.[26–28] The spread of pain may often occur in inflammatory conditions and peripheral injuries, which may produce enhancement of convergent afferent inputs to central nociceptive neurons. In addition, the convergence pattern may explain the theory of referred pain that is generated from toothache, headaches, temporomandibular disorders, sinusitis, and similar conditions.

Deafferentation and chronic pain

There may be some physiologic, neurochemical, and morphologic changes in somatosensory pathways involving the transmission of pain from the peripheral structures to the central nervous system. These phenomena may produce partial or total loss of sensory supply to and from a particular region of the body (see Fig 3-6). These conditions have been termed *deafferentation*. Although not fully explained, deafferentation may underlie the development of chronic orofacial pains.[23,29,30] This phenomenon induces sensory alterations that may be related to changes in the somatosensory pathways of the trigeminal nerve.

Fig 3-6 Central projection of the afferent system of the trigeminal nerve. The ophthalmic, maxillary, and mandibular branches of the trigeminal nerve enter the trigeminal ganglion (TG) synapse with the neurons of the substantia gelatinosa in the spinal nucleus of the fifth nerve (SN). The numbers represent the positions of the synaptic gate in cephalad (1), intermediary (2), and caudal locations (3). This arrangement explains the significance of facial lamination in cases of referred pains. Fibers from both sides of the face transit through the bulbar-thalamic tract (BT) to the thalamus (T) synapse in the posterior ventral nucleus (PVT) and medial nucleus (MT). From the thalamus, those nuclei send afferent projections to the paracentral cortex (PC) and orbitofrontal cortex (OF). At the level of the bulbar-thalamic tract, some projections of the afferent system go through the reticular formation (R), limbic system, and hypothalamus (H), and represent the affective component of the pain experience at the level of the orbitofrontal cortex.

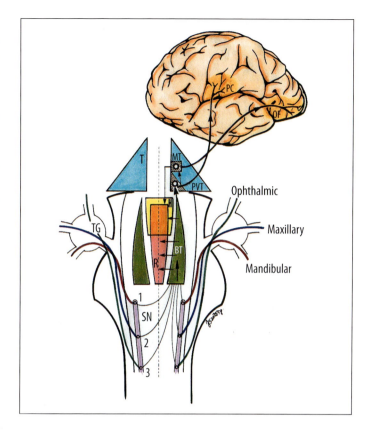

Some recent theories about chronic pain consider that alterations in the somatosensory pathways may produce localized organic changes in the structures of the central nervous system. This process may be initiated by trauma, compression, or degeneration of the nerve, which may lead to painful conditions such as trigeminal neuralgia, atypical facial neuralgia, and other forms of temporomandibular disorder.

MAXILLOFACIAL PAIN FROM SPECIFIC SOURCES

The remainder of this chapter presents a description of the most commonly encountered pain syndromes as a foundation for identification of pain in the maxillofacial region. Because pain mechanisms are still not totally understood, the following descriptions do not always apply in reproducible cause-effect relationships. Clinically speaking, some pain syndromes may be representative of the previously described phenomena, while others, although presenting the same clinical symptoms, may have a totally different etiology. Furthermore, all efforts must be directed to differentiate between chronic and acute pains.[31–35]

Some clinical conditions described in this chapter will be classified according to the pain source. Some of them will be manageable by a dental practitioner; however, others may need medical attention. An interprofessional consultation sometimes may be necessary in more complex cases.

Peripheral structures

The most common of all varieties of maxillofacial problems are dental and periodontal pains.[36]

Direct noxious stimulation or irritation to the following areas will lead to symptoms of facial pain of cutaneous, mucosal, and periosteal origin:

1. The skin covering the face by trauma (contusion, laceration, burning, etc) or infection (abscesses and cellulitis)
2. The mucous membrane covering the oral cavity, nose, or sinuses by infective lesions (eg, sinusitis or nasal infections)
3. The periosteum covering the facial skeleton as the result of fractures or osteomyelitis

These pains may be intensified by psychological conditions such as fear or oral fixation. In this situation, even light touch on the skin and/or any common functional activity in the area may become painful because of a lack of central inhibitory influences.

Muscles

This category of pain involves mainly skeletal muscles near the masticatory system, face, and neck. Pain from this source has a dull and steady quality. Although confined to facial structures, it is diffused, difficult to localize, and produces annoying sensations in the area. Sometimes when a muscle is activated, distorted, or stretched, this background sensation may become piercing pain.

The source of muscle pain is not totally known; however, some pain may be the result of irritation to the perivascular nerve plexuses in the adventitia of the blood vessels within the muscles. This irritation may be the consequence of exposure to abnormal concentrations of muscle metabolites, as a result of excessive and unaccustomed use.[37]

Pain may be caused by hyperactivity of the muscle, leading to fatigue. It has been shown that psychological or physical stress experienced by individuals may lead to increased activity of jaw muscles. Although many causes can be identified, the two most commonly encountered sources of muscle pain that may have special meaning in maxillofacial pain are muscle splinting and muscle spasm or trismus.

During the examination of muscle structures, tendons, and ligaments it is possible to distinguish some characteristics:

- Muscles present pain of slow conduction during rest. Pain sensations are dull. However, during action, the pain exhibits rapid transmission that is enhanced by contraction or passive distention (when the muscle mass is distorted).
- Tendons, ligaments, and fascia have pain of slow conduction during rest. Localization is clearly evident. There is a mechanism of self-protection leading to a pseudoparalysis. Sensitivity to touch is localized with precision.

Muscle splinting

Muscle splinting is characterized by the physiologic response arising from hyperactivity of certain muscles. This phenomenon produces limited movement and deviation of the mandible to protect injured teeth, muscles, and joints. Initiation of this muscle response (splinting) may be defined as a protective phenomenon where certain muscles involuntarily or reflexively (nociceptively and proprioceptively) contract to prevent the movement of an anatomic area or joint when injury or the threat of injury is perceived by the central nervous system.

Muscle splinting differs from muscle spasm in that the splinting muscle will relax when it does not have to protect another area and will even terminate its splinting action by resolution when the need for protection ceases. However, sustained splinting may develop into actual muscle spasm when contraction is sustained over an extended period of time.

Muscle spasm or trismus

Muscle spasm is characterized by sudden, involuntary contraction of one muscle or group of muscles, resulting in pain and usually interference with function. The contraction is sustained even when the muscle is at rest; therefore, the pain and dysfunction are present with passive as well as active movement of the structures involved.

A unique feature of muscle spasm pain is the phenomenon referred to as *cycling muscle spasm*, which often occurs in the masticatory region. This problem is characterized by the tendency of the muscle pain to perpetuate itself by generating painful impulses that result in excitatory reaction of the central nervous system.

This reaction cycles back to the spastic muscle, stimulating it again. As a result, other central excitatory effects may occur, thereby spreading pain to other regions.

Temporomandibular joint

Structures of the temporomandibular joint (TMJ) make a substantial contribution to the production of maxillofacial pain.[38–44] Mechanical or chemical irritation of peripheral pain receptors, which are related to the joint tissues, may lead directly to arthralgic pain. The nociceptive system (pain-conducting fibers) of the temporomandibular joint consists mainly of a dense plexus of unmyelinated, small-diameter, afferent, free-end nerve fibers that innervate throughout the fibrous capsule of the joint and bilaminar zone. Similar to the situation in other synovial joints, there are no nerve endings in the articular cartilage, meniscus, and synovial tissues of this joint; therefore, such structures are unable to produce any primary articular pain.

Pain experienced in the region of the temporomandibular joint arises mainly in these circumstances: the creation of abnormal mechanical stress in the fibrous capsule of the joint (possibly as a result of some form of malocclusion when the capsule or retrodiscal bilaminar zone is inflamed)[45–48] and the destruction of the articular surfaces by extensive degenerative disease.

Arthralgic pain can be described as a dull, depressing, nonlocalized discomfort of quite variable intensity. Eventually, it produces a sensation of warmth and can be aggravated by position and pressure. Movements in this case may produce lancinating pain.

The pressure-bearing portions (ie, articular surfaces and disc) have no receptors and therefore no afferent fibers whereby pain can be induced and transmitted to the central nervous system for perception. An exception is when rheumatoid arthritis is present.

The TMJ is a complex structure; therefore, several types of pain may emanate from the area, such as bone, tendon, ligament, fascia, muscle, synovial membrane, and blood vessel pain.

Vascular structures

This type of discomfort occurs more often than has been realized by either medical or dental professionals. It is evoked by mechanical or chemical irritation of the plexiform system of unmyelinated nerve fibers that are embedded in the adventitial sheaths of the blood vessels supplying the craniofacial tissues, mainly branches of the supraorbital, facial, and superficial temporal arteries (Fig 3-7).

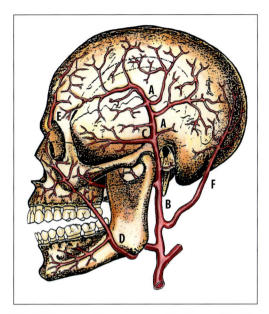

Fig 3-7 Branches of the external carotid artery supplying the head and neck. (A) Superficial temporal artery; (B) maxillary artery; (C) transverse facial artery; (D) facial artery; (E) supraorbital artery; (F) occipital artery. These branches are principal sectors of pain distribution in the face and head.

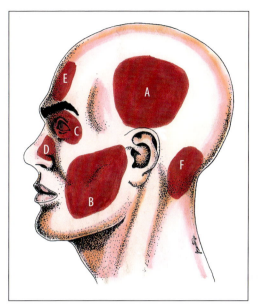

Fig 3-8 Areas of pain originating from craniofacial arteritis. (A, B, C, D) Pain from temporal arteritis; (E) pain from supraorbital arteritis; (F) pain from occipital arteritis.

Such irritations may occur in patients with vascular diseases, eg, arteriosclerosis or temporal arteritis (Fig 3-8), which is well recognized by competent physicians. Much more often, however, this pain results from episodic excessive dilation of blood vessels, such as in the case of migraine headaches (Fig 3-9). That is, when mechanically distorted, these blood vessels noxiously stimulate sensory receptors and afferent fibers within the vascular and perivascular tissues. Vascular pains have an annoying throbbing quality and are frequently accompanied by sensation of nausea and autonomic effects such as lacrimation and eye sensitivity to light. It is quite diffuse in location.

Clinical inspection is completely misleading as far as a neurologic model of localization is concerned, because vascular tree arborization (where the pain is felt) crosses other neurologic boundaries.

Neurologic disturbance

Maxillofacial pains that arise from some sort of neurologic disturbance have some characteristics in common. The quality of pain is intense and stimulating with a

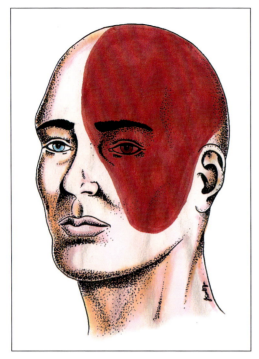

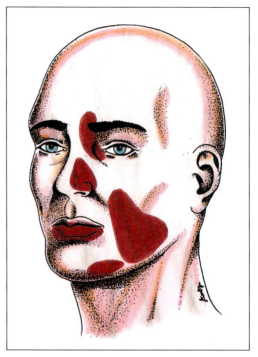

Fig 3-9 Craniofacial pain area affected by migraine headache.

Fig 3-10 Painful sectors on the orofacial regions arising from trigeminal neuralgia.

burning sensation. These types of pain are easily localized by the patient, considering the neuroanatomic distribution of the nerve trunks. The relationship between the stimulus and the response is always nonproportional and occasionally much more intense than the stimulus applied. In general, the most significant neuropathies encountered in clinical practice are:

- Neuromas: a disorganized mass of nervous tissue
- Scar tissue: formed following a surgical or accidental nerve amputation
- Neuritis: inflammation of sensory fibers
- Herpes zoster: neuritic involvement of the ganglion, sensory root, or medullary tract of a nerve by the chicken pox virus
- Trigeminal neuralgia: idiopathic neuralgia that includes changes in the fibers of the ganglion and dorsal root; its precise etiology is not known[49] (Fig 3-10)

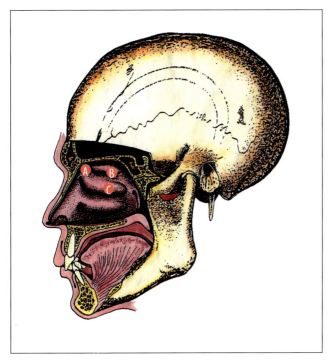

Fig 3-11 Sinus structures. (A) Ethmoid sinus; (B) superior turbinate; (C) middle turbinate.

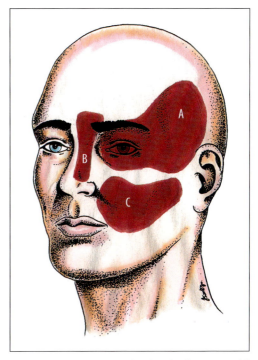

Fig 3-12 Sinus pain areas referred to facial structures. (A) Pain referred from the ethmoid sinus; (B) pain referred from the superior turbinate; (C) pain referred from the middle turbinate.

REFERRED MAXILLOFACIAL PAIN

Pain may be referred to maxillofacial regions from different structures, mainly:

- Mucosal tissues of the nose and paranasal sinuses, where afferent projections from their sensory receptor systems converge synaptically on neurons in the spinal nucleus of the trigeminal nerve (Figs 3-11 and 3-12).
- Groups of maxillary and mandibular teeth where regions of the face, innervated by the mandibular and maxillary branches of the fifth nerve, may be diffusely painful. Some masticatory muscles may also present some form of dysfunction, which will be capable of referring poorly localized pain to teeth and orofacial-structures (Figs 3-13 and 3-14). Sometimes, due to its intensity, this kind of pain can be easily confused with trigeminal neuralgia; for this reason, it is known as *atypical facial neuralgia*.

- Myogenic origin involving the masticatory and cervical muscles, where trigger mechanisms (located in the body of a given muscle) may produce discomfort in zones of pain reference on the face and head (Figs 3-15 to 3-22). In this category of pain, it is very common for muscle tension headaches to occur (Fig 3-23), complicating the analysis of craniomandibular symptoms.
- Temporomandibular arthropathies. Inherent pain and dysfunction as a result of these arthropathies may produce secondary myalgia and muscle spasm so that the area of complaint in the maxillofacial region may be considerably larger than the site of origin (Fig 3-24). The overall problem may represent the chief complaint of the patient, or the condition may remain subacute and not be discovered until palpation or provocation tests are performed. Pain is elicited at rest, on movement, or both. It is very important to ascertain whether it is an intrinsic pain (using a provocative test with separator) or a pain referred from muscles, teeth (pulp test), or heart. Painful stimulation of the joint structures typically induces predominant contraction of flexor muscles. Free nerve endings, which are common in joint capsule, may be activated by vigorous twisting or stretching of the capsule (which may occur during extreme bruxing movements).
- Vascular origin. In this case, it is also common to have the combination of secondary central excitatory effects. The vascular component of mastication and neck muscle pain is the most significant one and has been considered the main source for myalgia. Areas of reference on the head and face, together with complex symptoms of masticatory pain and dysfunction, are frequently developed as a result of secondary pain induced by vascular problems.

It is imperative that the clinician be familiar with various biologic mechanisms and concepts pertaining to head and neck musculature, to diagnose and treat many functional disturbances associated with the masticatory system. In particular, from an occlusion standpoint, the professional should be aware of the complex role played by the musculature in the anatomic and physiologic interaction among various components (teeth, muscles, joints, etc). In addition, there may be intervening actions in muscle function from conscious and unconscious emotional sources.

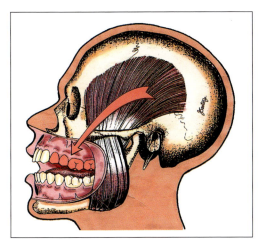

Fig 3-13 Atypical facial neuralgia. Some masticatory muscles may refer pain to the maxillary teeth, for example, pain referred from the anterior, middle, and posterior bundles of the temporalis muscle *(arrow)*.

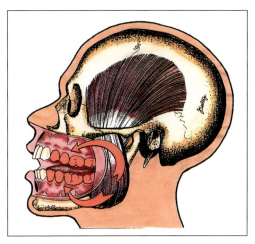

Fig 3-14 Atypical facial neuralgia. The masseter muscle also has potential to refer pain to the mandibular and maxillary teeth *(arrows)*.

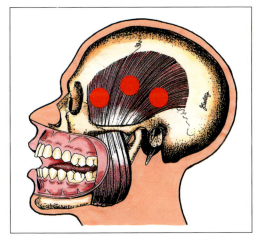

Fig 3-15 Temporalis muscle. *Red dots* represent areas where primary pain may be felt.

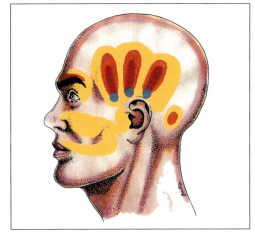

Fig 3-16 Areas of superficial pain referred to the face and head from the temporalis muscle. In this drawing and Figs 3-18 to 3-24, the intensity of the color is in proportion to the intensity of the pain, and the *blue dots* indicate trigger points.

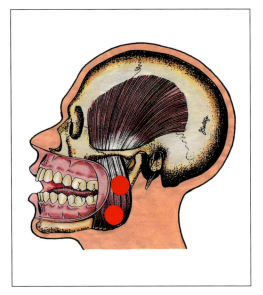

Fig 3-17 Masseter muscle. *Red dots* represent the possible location where primary pain is felt.

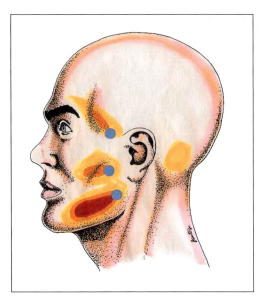

Fig 3-18 Craniofacial pain referred from the superficial portion of the masseter muscle.

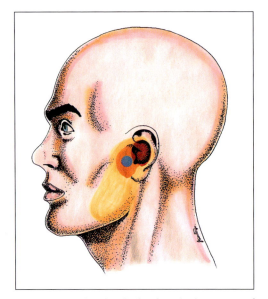

Fig 3-19 Pain referred to the face from the deep portion of the masseter muscle. Note the intensity of pain in the regions of the temporomandibular joint and ear.

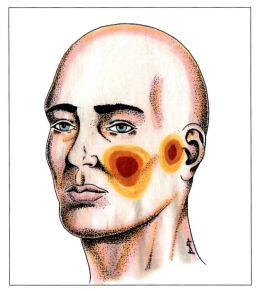

Fig 3-20 Pain referred to the face from the lateral pterygoid muscle. The trigger point is located intraorally.

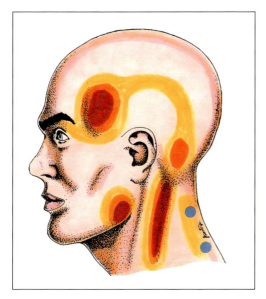

Fig 3-21 Craniofacial superficial pain referred from the trapezius muscle.

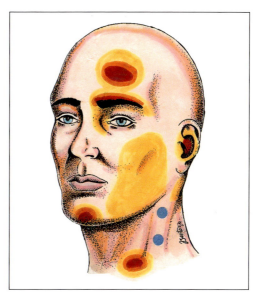

Fig 3-22 Zones of referred pain from the sternocleidomastoid muscle. Note the intensity of pain felt in the auricular area.

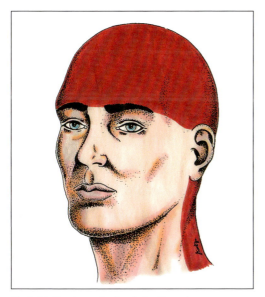

Fig 3-23 Muscle tension headache. The red area represents the vise-cap location of the diffuse pain, accompanied by tightness, pressure, and, occasionally, throbbing pain.

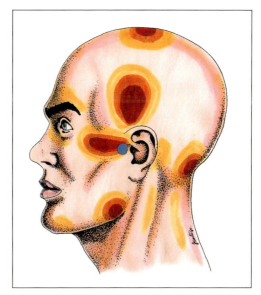

Fig 3-24 Facial areas of pain referred from the temporomandibular joint.

MAXILLOFACIAL PAIN OF PSYCHOLOGICAL ORIGIN

Pain in its psychological aspect is an experience, which proves the involvement of the psyche and the soma. Thus, the psychosomatic aspect of pain is inseparable from the physical. The term *pain experience* has been suggested as an alternative to *pain*, because it includes the individual's integration of all the effects of noxious stimuli, including the reactions to pain threat, physical sensations, and physiologic reaction. Other sociological factors, such as beliefs attributed to pain, the age of the patient, and ethnic background, seem to contribute to the pain response.

MAXILLOFACIAL PAIN ASSOCIATED WITH NAUSEA AND VOMITING

Craniomandibular disorders may induce nausea and vomiting (emetic symptoms).[52] In general, patients distressed with disorders in the internal portion of the TMJ complain of otalgia, headache, discomfort in the preauricular area, and pain behind the eyes, neck, shoulders, and arms. Other manifestations may include vertigo, tachycardia, bruxism, and digestive problems. In these cases, patients with bruxism mostly exhibit not tooth grinding but tooth clenching behavior. Unfortunately, cases of bruxism that involve only clenching tend to be difficult to diagnose.

The connections between masticatory system parafunction and nausea and vomiting are related to projections of the spinal nucleus of the trigeminal nerve inside the nucleus tractus solitarius (NTS), including also projections of the facial (VII interpolaris), glossopharyngeal (IX), and vagus (X) sensory nerves into this same nucleus (Fig 3-25). Therefore, it has been identified that the trigeminal nerve is not the only source of sensory projections to the brain stem. The NTS at the level of the obex is the main site to which messages from both the area postrema and peripheral afferents are transmitted. This nucleus is, consequently, a presumable candidate for the location of interactions between the area postrema and peripheral afferent signals (see Fig 3-25). The NTS is recognized as the chief conveyor of the peripheral cardiovascular, respiratory, and gastrointestinal apparatus.

Furthermore, intense substance P–like immunoreactivity is observed in bundles of fibers passing between the spinal nucleus of the trigeminal nerve and the ventral-lateral NTS, which are adjacent to the area postrema. The presence of a trigeminal solitary projection, which is composed of trigeminal sensory neurons

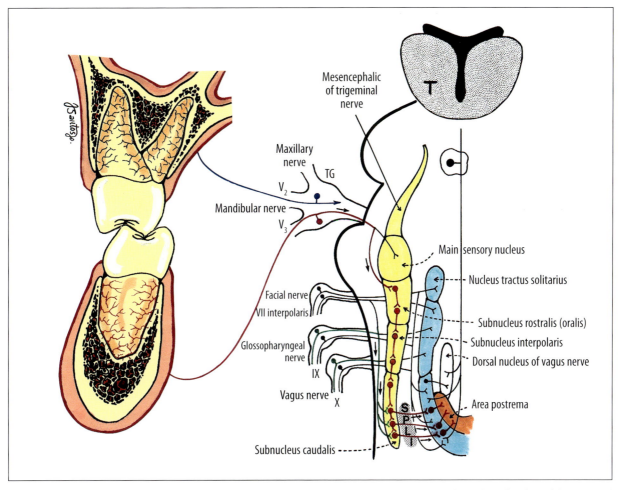

Fig 3-25 Connections between masticatory system parafunction (clenching) and nausea and vomiting at the level of spinal nucleus of the trigeminal nerve inside the nucleus of the solitary tract. (SPLI) Substance P–like immunoreactivity; (T) thalamus; (TG) trigeminal ganglion.

containing substance P, suggests an anatomic pathway whereby this same substance P may modulate vagal or glossopharyngeal sensory information.

During the day, some patients clench their teeth with moderate intensity of force. However, the nocturnal clenching during sleep may exert considerable force. In some cases, upon waking, patients describe feelings of fatigue and affliction from nausea and/or vomiting. Moreover, periodontal mechanoreceptors present projections to the hypothalamus; in this circumstance, most of the periodontal mechanoreceptors are prone to stimulate the area postrema, directly via the NTS and secondarily via the hypothalamus by means of the dorsal longitudinal tractus, when clenching occurs. At the level of the hypothalamus, periodontal afferents may either produce emetic reactions or inhibit the activity of hypothalamic cells.

MAXILLOFACIAL PAIN RESULTING FROM WHIPLASH INJURIES

In automotive impacts, injuries at the level of the cervical column and the articulation of maxillary bones are the result of intense inertial acceleration.[51-54] The increase of vehicles in urban areas, combined with the irresponsibility and lack of ability of some drivers, causes considerable incidence of these accidents.

Whiplash injuries are the result of rear collisions between vehicles. They occur, in the majority of cases, when a target vehicle is stopped at a street intersection waiting for a traffic light to change and another automobile (bullet vehicle) collides from behind. These collisions may occur at low speeds (10 to 30 mph) or even at medium speeds (40 to 60 mph).

The inertial acceleration imparted to the target vehicle, at the moment of the impact, produces a quick backward oscillation of the head, or hyperextension, followed by an immediate compensatory forward movement, or hyperflexion (Fig 3-26). This oscillation occurs in milliseconds and, in the majority of the cases, the victim is not prepared to react to the blow produced by the acceleration. This rapid action is described as a *whiplash lesion* to nerves and neural ganglia and involves pinching of the spinal ganglion because of intervertebral compression. Plasmatic leakage through the neural membrane may also occur. Distant symptoms may arise in areas of sensitive neural segments. This phenomenon is the result of regional divisions in the body (dermatomes) that are located distant to the area of injury.

Dental professionals must be concerned with this type of event. Injuries resulting from these accidents may produce serious complications in the head, face, masticatory apparatus, and neck. Although such injuries may not be considered the main source for the onset of temporomandibular dysfunction, an accident involving the collision of automotive vehicles may produce later pain symptoms from reflex influences starting at the victim's cervical column. These reflex pains generate secondary painful and dysfunctional components in the temporomandibular joints, masticatory muscles, cervical nerves (which are responsible for the motor and sensitive innervations of the masticatory apparatus), and other structures. An individual with these problems will complain to the clinician about difficulty in mastication, increased limitation of mouth opening, joint locking, constant muscle fatigue, pain around the facial structures, cephalgia, and other problems.

Some vehicles have plastic physical characteristics (ie, deform easily), while others have elasticity (with low tendency to deformation). Vehicle weights are important factors. A light and plastic target vehicle, when receiving the impact from a heavy and elastic one, will suffer too much deformation. The target vehicle will absorb, at the moment of the impact, a great deal of kinetic energy that is produced by the bullet vehicle.

The effect duration of a collision impact does not go beyond 175 milliseconds, which plays a part in the acceleration imparted to the occupants of the vehicles.

Fig 3-26 Hyperextension and hyperflexion of the head.

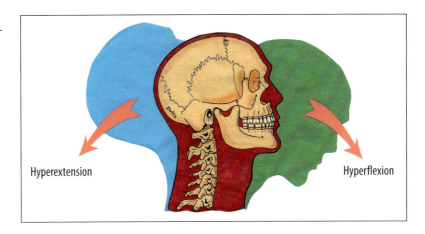

Fig 3-27 Oscillation of the head during the impact.

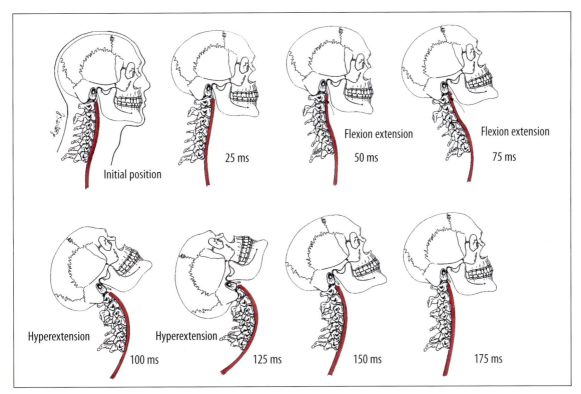

The most critical phase, ie, when most of lesions may occur, is around 125 milliseconds, because the head oscillates violently.

If the collision is unexpected, the occupant of the target vehicle will have minimal ability to react to the impact, because the human neuromuscular reflex system (myotatic reflex) takes about 500 milliseconds to complete (Fig 3-27). If the impact is anticipated, the most usual action of both vehicles' occupants is to prepare, tensing

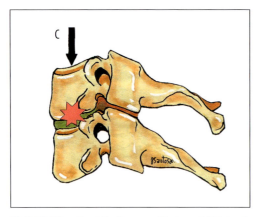

Fig 3-28 When the victim is prepared for impact, high bending stresses are followed by compressive forces (C) from the neck muscles, which limit the bending. Whiplash injury includes high pressure in the center of the intervertebral discs and damage to the vertebral body and end plates.

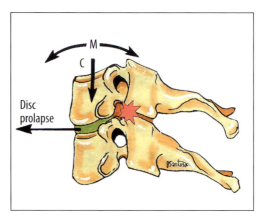

Fig 3-29 When the collision is only partially anticipated by the victim, the neck muscles are not able to hold the head steady, and bending moments (M) and compressive forces (C) act at the same time. Whiplash injury occurs as the central part of the disc is pressurized and displaced through the stretched and weakened annulus.

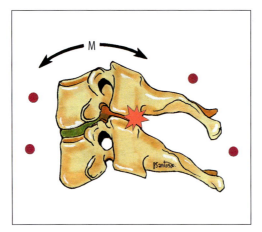

Fig 3-30 When the victim does not anticipate the collision, there is no protective muscle contraction to counteract the bending moments (M). Whiplash injury includes damage to muscles and ligaments far from the disc's center of rotation. *Red dots* represent damage to cervical structures distant from the vertebral center of rotation.

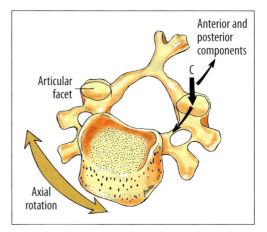

Fig 3-31 In a side-impact collision, there is lateral rotation of the vertebrae centered on the articular facets, causing high shearing stresses and subsequent laceration of the vertebral arteries and spinal nerve. (C) Compressive forces.

the neck by contracting cervical and shoulder muscles. At the impact, forces capable of producing oscillatory movements of the head are compensated for by strong compressive tensions, because of the contraction of cervical muscles. Although injuries are less extensive, the increased pressure at the center of vertebrae can produce rupture of intervertebral cervical disks and probable damage to the vertebral body (Fig 3-28).

Fig 3-32 Cervical spinal cord. The cervical branches of the cervical nerves C2 and C3 join the spinal accessory nerve to the sternocleidomastoid and trapezius muscles.

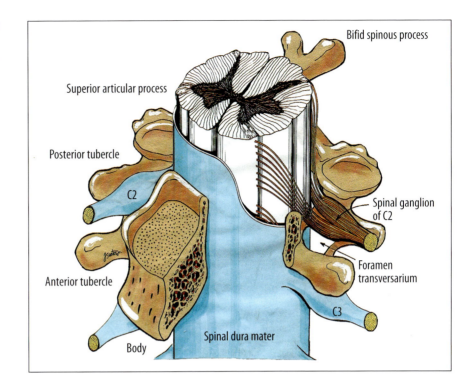

If collision is only partially anticipated, the occupants of both vehicles are able to prepare for the impact almost at the exact moment of the event. In this case, the shoulder and neck musculature are not able to maintain the stability of the head. Bascule forces and compressive tensions are acting simultaneously. The central portion of the intervertebral disc will be compressed, with the ensuing displacement of the anterior portion of the disc (disc prolapse) at the level of the anterior borders of the vertebrae (Fig 3-29).

When the collision is unexpected, mainly by the occupant of the target vehicle, there will probably be no protective contraction of the shoulder and neck muscles (Fig 3-30). Bascule movements will dominate the displacement of the head, overpowering compressive tensions. In these conditions, besides injuries concentrated in the vertebrae and intervertebral discs, there will be direct action against muscles and ligaments located distant to vertebral centers of rotation.

If the collision occurs on the lateral portion of the target vehicle, there will be rotation of the cervical vertebrae of the occupant as a result of sudden rotation of the head. These torque tensions present shearing forces of high intensity and have a tendency to damage the structures inside and around the vertebrae. Consequently, the dominant axial rotation imparted to the head will produce lacerations to the vertebral arteries and the spinal nerve. This type of collision is more damaging to victims than the direct posterior impact (Fig 3-31).

Figures 3-32 to 3-36 illustrate some aspects of whiplash injury affecting cervical areas of the body. Surgical procedures that can be used in the treatment of

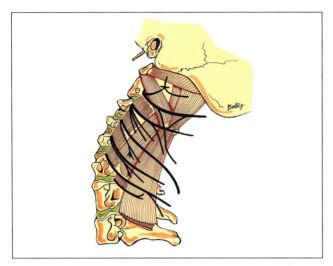

Fig 3-33 Whiplash injury with damage to the spinal ganglion and nerves. Lesions to nerves and nervous ganglions may pinch the spinal nerve because of intervertebral compression. The result may be evidence of plasma membrane leakage, symptoms in areas of dermatomes, disruption of nerve functions, proprioceptive muscle dysfunction, blurring of vision and ocular pain, headaches, tinnitus, and dizziness with or without vertigo. Section of nerves.

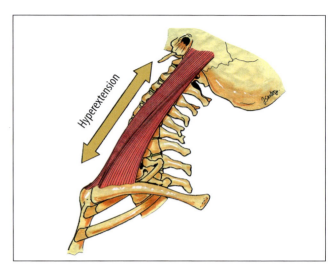

Fig 3-34 Effects of whiplash injury associated with the sternocleidomastoid muscle include stretching and tearing of musculature, tenderness, dizziness, interference with neck-uprighting reflexes, interference with postural control system, and muscle spasm.

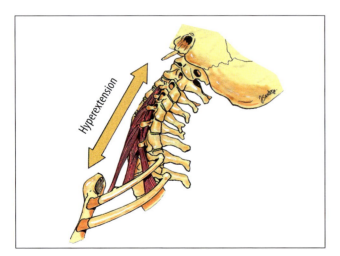

Fig 3-35 Effects of whiplash injury associated with the scalenus muscle include spasm and thickening of fibers and tendency to spasm, rigidity, and hypertrophy or even hypotrophy of facial and cervical muscles. The postural position of the head and the patient will be altered due to these problems. If there is compression of the brachial plexus, the patient may experience difficult oxygenation during sleep, scalenus anticus syndrome, or carpal tunnel syndrome. There will be impairment of the head and mandible.

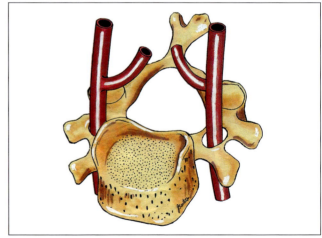

Fig 3-36 Effects of whiplash injury associated with damage to the vertebral artery. There may be compression and occlusion of arteries localized at the level of the vertebrae. Further, there will be the onset of muscular alterations and fibroid changes along cranial nerve pathways. Some patients may suffer stroke or acute chronic ischemia of the brain stem and occipital lobes.

whiplash injury include neurotomy (electrocoagulation of vertebral nerves at the level of the ganglion) through direct application of electric currents and surgical placement of metallic implants in and/or around the cervical vertebrae.

OBSTRUCTIVE SLEEP APNEA

Obstructive sleep apnea (OSA)[55,56] is defined as cessation of breathing or airflow for periods of 10 seconds or more. It is called obstructive because airflow ceases despite continued respiratory chest (thoracic-abdominal wall activity) and diaphragm movement (electromyographic activity). During apnea, breathing becomes labored and noisy. Patients with this syndrome present with an apnea index greater than or equal to five episodes per hour (in some cases, an apnea index as high as 10 may be normal, depending on age), an apnea/hypopnea index greater than or equal to 10, and excessive daytime sleepiness.

The syndrome is caused by an unfavorable anatomic configuration in the pharyngeal airway. This unfavorable pharyngeal anatomy causes collapse of the airway walls when negative pressure is exerted during inspiration. The dimensions and configuration of the skull base, vertebral column, maxilla, and mandible establish the shape and volume of the three-dimensional space in the pharyngeal soft structures (tongue, soft palate, faucial tonsils, and posterior pharyngeal walls)[57,58] (Fig 3-37).

Obstruction of the airway is thought to be caused by the occlusion of the pharynx as the tongue settles back (posteriorly) against the pharyngeal wall. The cause is presumed to be gravitational influences on the tongue and soft palate against the unmovable pharyngeal wall (see Fig 3-37).

Significant changes in oral pharyngeal airflow characteristics arise with a change in body position from upright to supine and mandibular position from normal to protrusive. Airflow capacity may be returned to normal by moving the jaw forward while in supine position.

Complications

Patients with OSA commonly exhibit systemic hypertension. Patients will complain of morning headache[26–28] and/or present with a cardiac arrhythmia. Daytime somnolence varies from mild (falling asleep while watching TV) to severe (falling asleep during conversation). A complete medical evaluation is necessary as part of the

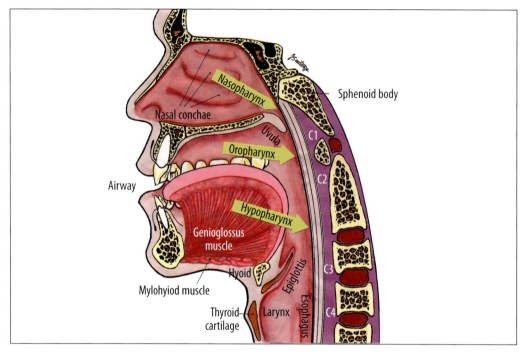

Fig 3-37 Anatomic structures usually involved in sleep apnea.

workup for the complaint of daytime sleepiness. Patients with OSA also have an increased incidence of cerebrovascular accidents.

Some patients experience intermittent cessation of breathing or other respiratory diseases. In these cases, the patient should be screened for diabetes, hypothyroidism, and cardiovascular problems. Obesity is a significant factor in OSA, and weight control and counseling are sometimes recommended as conservative first steps in the management of OSA. Death can result from occlusion of the airway.

Diagnosis

Polysomnography is the most widely accepted procedure for diagnostic confirmation of apneas. This test is able to define the respiratory disturbance index, which refers to the number of apnea/hypopnea episodes (oxygen desaturation greater than 4%) per hour on a polysomnograph. As standard protocol, 16-channel polysomnography recordings are simultaneously integrated with closed-circuit infrared television monitoring, which permits visual observation in case the patient experiences respiratory distress. Overnight polysomnography is used to confirm the diagnosis, providing multiple recordings of respiratory functions.

After the pretreatment polysomnography, the patient may undergo magnetic resonance imaging of the TMJ and upper airway.

Polysomnography features the integration of the following parameters:

- Central and occipital electroencephalograms
- Right and left electro-oculogram/eye movement
- Digastric (submental) and tibialis electromyogram
- Heart rate and rhythm electrocardiogram
- Oronasal inhalation/exhalation airflow (right and left nares and mouth); continuous airflow assessment by an oronasal three-way temperature thermistor
- Respiratory effort (abdominal, ribcage movement); chest wall excursions by thoracic and abdominal impedance plethysmography
- Oxygen desaturation pulse (oxyhemoglobin saturation measurements) or finger oximetry
- Body position
- Breathing sounds
- Motor activity of extremity movements

Health care team

Treatment of OSA is best accomplished in coordination with the medical staff consultant and should not be done solely by the dental team. Both teams work together in the best interest of the individual patients and their treatment needs. A lack of physician involvement can lead to failure to recognize and treat medical sequelae of OSA, such as hypertension, or the failure to recognize other underlying systemic diseases (pulmonary or cardiovascular), which may be mistakenly treated as OSA.

Clinicians have been criticized for demedicalizing sleep-disordered breathing. Otolaryngologists and pulmonary specialists have been questioned about their prescription of home monitoring systems and self-titrating continuous positive air pressure (CPAP) devices; opponents argue that these decisions toward home care are despecializing the treatment of sleep-disordered breathing, which should be treated by a multidisciplinary team.

Surgical treatment modalities

There is no single surgical procedure that will eliminate OSA. The option of a surgical approach for the treatment of OSA must be thoroughly investigated prior to commitment, with the understanding (by physician and patient) that some surgeries are successful and others may result in failures.

The commitment to a surgical approach may require an establishment of a surgical team: otorhinolaryngologist, maxillofacial surgeon, and bariatric surgeon.

Uvulopalatopharyngoplasty

Uvulopalatopharyngoplasty (UPPP), a treatment modality used to enlarge pharyngeal air space, has only a 50% success rate.[59] Surgery involves excision of soft tissue (palate, uvula, tonsils, and posterior/lateral pharyngeal wall), and trimming and reorientation of the anterior and posterior tonsil pillars. If the obstruction is located below the oropharynx, surgery is contraindicated. Documented complications include postoperative stenosis, significant postoperative pain, infection, nasal regurgitation, velopharyngeal insufficiency for more than 1 month, postoperative bleeding, nasopharyngeal stenosis, voice change, and a vague foreign-body sensation. The morbidity rate for UPPP is quite high.

Laser-assisted uvulopalatoplasty

Laser-assisted uvulopalatoplasty (LAUP), a procedure used to resculpture the soft palate, is less invasive than UPPP. The retropalatal airway is enlarged by ablation of the uvula and posterior margin of the soft palate with a carbon dioxide laser; the procedure does not include ablation of the tonsil area. It can be done under local anesthesia in a physician's office; the surgery is usually applied as a treatment for snoring without presence of OSA. In the long term, LAUP may result in diminished velopharyngeal space and therefore is contraindicated for OSA.

Anterior-inferior mandibular osteotomy

Anterior-inferior mandibular osteotomy (AIMO) consists of detachment of the mylohyoid muscle and stretching of the geniohyoid, genioglossal, and digastric muscles. This stretching should achieve permanent advancement of the hyoid bone and thereby also the base of the tongue. The failure of AIMO to have a positive effect on OSA might be explained by an adaptation within the suprahyoid and posthyoid muscle complex soon after the surgery. The adaptation results in an almost unchanged position of the hyoid bone and the tongue. Hence, the airway space is not widened by the surgical procedure.

Maxillomandibular advancement

Maxillomandibular advancement (MMA) provides maximal enlargement of the retrolingual airway. The maxilla and mandible are advanced simultaneously by means of Le Fort I maxillary and sagittal split mandibular osteotomies, allowing the extreme degree of mandibular advancement that is required to treat OSA. Patients must be evaluated carefully to determine if they are candidates for the procedure, because MMA results in mandibular prognathism. Patients with OSA, maxillomandibular deficiency, dolichofacial characteristics, and narrow retrolingual airway space are treated with success, but an increased risk of morbidity is involved with progressive surgical procedures.

Nonsurgical treatment modalities

Continuous positive air pressure

Continuous positive air pressure (CPAP) involves the wearing of a nasal mask over the nose during sleep; pressure from an air compressor forces air through nasal passages into the airway. This is a pneumatic splint used to hold the airway open at night with a 100% success rate. This may be the preferred form of treatment for severe respiratory distress and is currently considered the primary treatment for OSA. Since the 1980s, CPAP has been the most widely accepted conservative and traditional method for treatment of mild-to-moderate OSA. Although cumbersome under optimized clinical conditions, CPAP is a very effective, nonsurgical treatment option.

Patient compliance (only 35%) is a factor, because patients often cannot tolerate the nasal CPAP and therefore are creating a demand for an alternative, noninvasive treatment that is safe, effective, and acceptable. Only 50% to 80% of patients use this treatment on a long-term basis, and of these patients fewer than 50% use the CPAP at night. In conjunction with CPAP, medications may be used to modify nasopharyngeal edema and congestion (such as chronic rhinitis).

Mandibular-repositioning device

Mandibular-repositioning devices (MRDs) are major conservative treatment approaches to the complex problem of OSA.[60-63] By advancing the mandible, the anterior mandibular-repositioning device increases the airway caliber and decreases the airway resistance when worn during sleep. The goal for such therapy is to increase the airway patency. Oral appliances are either mandibular advancers or tongue advancers, both utilized to enlarge the upper airway. MRDs are available as many different oral appliances. The precise mode of action of these oral appliances is still to be determined; among the possibilities being considered are increased upper airway caliber, activation of upper airway dilator muscles (increase of pharyngeal and genioglossus muscle activity), decreased upper airway compliance, and stabilization of soft tissues, thus preventing airway collapse.

The use of a jaw-repositioning appliance for OSAs has been increasingly noticed in both dental and medical literature since the 1980s. The clinical role of these appliances warrants evaluation because of the need for an effective, low-risk alternative to CPAP. The American Sleep Disorder Association (ASDA) in 1995 stated that oral appliances should be a primary treatment option for patients with mild, moderate, and severe OSA who cannot tolerate treatment with CPAP. However, the role of oral appliances in the treatment of OSA may even be broader than that envisioned in ASDA practice parameters.

A wide variety of intraoral orthotic repositioning appliances have been advocated, and numerous designs have been described in the literature. The lack of standardization in the use of oral appliances for the treatment of OSA has been problematic. Not only do the oral appliances vary in design, specific mode of action, cost, and manufacturers, but practitioners vary in their pretreatment procedures, diagnostic workups, follow-up care, and tests.

MRDs are effective in more than half of patients with severe OSA, although most of the overall treatment failures were found in subgroups. No patients had developed chronic TMJ difficulties or any other complications as a result of MRD use. Although patients with severe OSA are likely to receive at least adequate treatment with an MRD, individual patients may have dramatic treatment responses. Daytime sleepiness also appears to improve subjectively with MRD treatment. It appears that MRDs are a second-line therapy in patients with severe OSA, resulting in a treatment response approximating that obtained with UPPP.[58,60–62]

It is unknown whether the effect of an MRD on apneas differs between patients who have apneas predominantly in the supine sleep position and those who have apneas in other sleep positions. A tongue-retaining device is more efficient at reducing the frequency of apnea experienced in the supine position than it is in the lateral sleep position. Apneas are found more frequently in patients sleeping in the supine position, probably due to the gravitation influence to the mandible and tongue.

Objective posttreatment testing is very important in assessing the efficacy of an oral appliance. The effects of mandibular advancement may vary from almost complete elimination of apneas in some patients to the presence of apneas in other patients. The success is greater in patients with mild OSA than in those with moderate-to-severe cases. The causes of the differences are unknown. Efficacy is based on the appliance's ability to reposition the jaw and bring the tongue and accompanying soft tissues of the pharynx forward.

A study of MRDs reported that mandibular protrusion ranged from 7 to 10 mm.[61] Serial adjustment was 1 to 2 mm. Forward positioning of the mandible and downward placement of the mandible (8 mm) coincided with a decrease in apnea

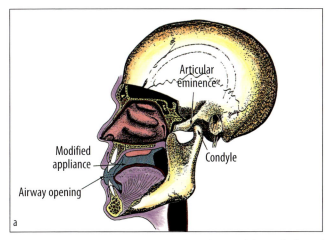
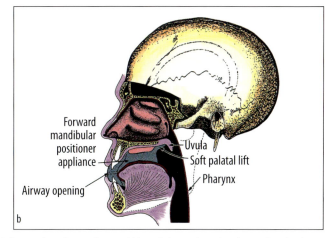

Fig 3-38 Mandibular-repositioning device (modification of the regular bite splint) designed to advance the mandible and elevate the soft palate and uvula, shown in sagittal naso-oropharyngeal sections with *(a)* and without *(b)* the mandible.

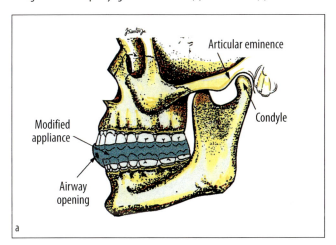
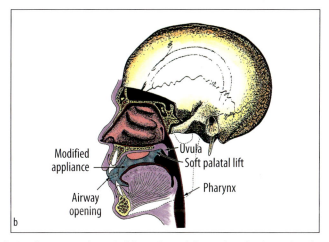

Fig 3-39 Mandibular-repositioning device (modification of the regular bite splint) designed to increase the vertical dimension and elevate the soft palate and uvula, shown in lateral view *(a)* and sagittal naso-oropharyngeal section *(b)*.

episodes from 29 to 19 per hour, and a reduction in respiratory disturbance index (apneic plus hypopneic) from 54 to 36 per hour. Cephalometric readings confirmed the increase in pharyngeal space.[61]

The majority of oral appliances require dental impressions, bite registration, and (often) laboratory fabrication in their construction. Some appliances are prefabricated and can be molded in the office to the patient's teeth. Some appliances restrict the mouth opening by means of clasps.

Some appliances feature a posterior extension of the maxillary component to modify the position of the soft palate or tongue (Figs 3-38 and 3-39). Other oral appliances feature progressive repositioning of the mandible after initial delivery.

Mandibular advancement oral appliances require at least 10 teeth in both the maxillary and mandibular arches. Movement also includes downward rotation of the mandible.

Other types include a tongue retainer that keeps the tongue in an anterior position during sleep by means of negative pressure on a soft plastic bulb. This tongue-retaining device is available in both custom-fabricated and prefabricated versions and can be used for edentulous patients.

Dental appliances are quite effective and less invasive than surgical intervention.

MRD versus CPAP

- MRD has fewer side effects. It may be preferred by patients.
- CPAP is tolerated by patients with more severe OSA, whereas the MRD is well tolerated by patients with mild and moderate OSA.
- Psychosocial issues may prevent individual patients from complying with CPAP use. These issues include inconvenience for patients who travel frequently, lack of acceptance by bedpartners, and stigmatization of patients living in communal conditions such as military barracks.

REFERENCES

1. Association Reports. Report of the President's conference on the examination, diagnosis and management of TMJ disorders. J Am Dent Assoc 1983;106:75–77.
2. Bell WE. Temporomandibular Disorders: Classification, Diagnosis, Management, ed 3. Chicago: Year Book Medical, 1990.
3. Bell WE. Orofacial Pains: Classification, Diagnosis, Management, ed 4. Chicago: Year Book Medical, 1989.
4. Breault MR. Eagle's syndrome: Review of the literature and implications in craniomandibular disorders. Cranio 1986;4:323–337.
5. Clark GT, Solberg WK (eds). Perspectives in Temporomandibular Disorders. Chicago: Quintessence, 1987.
6. de Laat A. Scientific basis of masticatory disorders. In: Lindsen RWA (ed). Frontiers of Oral Biology. Vol 9: The scientific basis of eating. New York: Karger, 1998:122–134.
7. dos Santos J Jr, Murakami T, Nelson SJ. Orthopedic considerations of the cervical syndrome and temporomandibular disorders. Tex Dent J 1989;106(11):8–13.
8. Farrar WB, McCarthy WL Jr. A Clinical Outline of TMJ Diagnosis and Treatment, ed 7. Montgomery, AL: Normandy, 1982.
9. Report of the President's Conference on the Examination, Diagnosis, and Management of Temporomandibular Disorders. J Am Dent Assoc 1983;106:75–77.
10. Jendrensen MD, Allen EP, Bayne SC, et al. Annual review of selected dental literature: Report of the Committee on Scientific Investigation of the American Academy of Restorative Dentistry. J Prosthet Dent 1994;72:39–40.

11. Kerr DA, Ash MM, Millard HD. Oral Diagnosis, ed 6. St Louis: Mosby, 1983.

12. Kraus SL. TMJ Disorders: Management of the Craniomandibular Complex. New York: Churchill Livingstone, 1988.

13. Le Resche L, Truelove EL, Dworkin SF. Temporomandibular disorders: A survey of dentists' knowledge and beliefs. J Am Dent Assoc 1993;124:90–105.

14. American Academy of Orofacial Pain. Management. In: McNeill C (ed). Temporomandibular Disorders. Guidelines for Classification, Assessment, and Management. Chicago: Quintessence, 1993:81–107.

15. Moses AJ. Scientific methodology in temporomandibular disorders. 3. Diagnostic reasoning. Cranio 1994;12;259–265.

16. Okeson JP. Management of Temporomandibular Disorders, ed 3. St Louis: Mosby Year Book, 1993.

17. Okeson JP. Orofacial Pain: Guidelines for Assessment, Diagnosis, and Management. Chicago: Quintessence, 1996.

18. Parker MW. A dynamic model of etiology in temporomandibular disorders. J Am Dent Assoc 1990;120:283–290.

19. Pullinger AG, Seligman DA, Gornbein JA. A multiple logistic regression analysis of the risk and relative odds of temporomandibular disorders as a function of common occlusal factors. J Dent Res 1993;72:968–979.

20. Rusiecki RS. Chest pain as a result of temporomandibular disorder (TMD). Gen Dent 1998; 46:352–355.

21. Swerdlow M, Charlton JE. Relief of Intractable Pain, ed 4. Amsterdam: Elsevier, 1989.

22. Tegelberg A, Kopp S. Short-term effect of physical training on TMJ disorder in individuals with rheumatoid arthritis and ankylosis spondylitis. Acta Odontol Scand 1988;46:49–56.

23. Aronoff GM. Evaluation and Treatment of Chronic Pain, ed 2. Baltimore: Williams & Wilkins, 1992.

24. Ash MM, Ramfjord SP. Occlusion, ed 4. Philadelphia: Saunders, 1995.

25. Travell JC, Simons DG. Myofascial Pain and Dysfunction. The Trigger Points Manual. Baltimore: Williams & Wilkins, 1983.

26. Bailey DR. Tension headache and bruxism in sleep disordered patients. Cranio 1990;8:174–182.

27. Diamond S, Dalessio DJ. The Practicing Physician's Approach to Headache, ed 5. Baltimore: Williams & Wilkins, 1992.

28. Graham JR. Headache. In: Aronoff GM (ed). Evaluation and Treatment of Chronic Pain. Baltimore: Urban & Schwartzenberg, 1985.

29. Hendler NH. Diagnosis and Treatment of Chronic Pain. Boston: Wright, 1982:193–199,201–210.

30. Turner JA, Chapman CR. Psychological interventions for chronic pain: A critical review. Relaxation training and biofeedback. Pain 1982;12:1–21.

31. Dionne RA, Phero JC. Management of Pain and Anxiety in Dental Practice. New York: Elsevier, 1991.

32. Fields HL. Pain. New York: McGraw-Hill, 1987.

33. Lipton S, Miles J. Persistent Pain: Modern Methods of Treatment. London: Grune & Stratton, 1983.

34. Sessle BJ. Neural mechanisms of oral and facial pain. Otolaryngol Clin North Am 1989;22: 1059–1072.

35. Stohler CS, Ashton-Miller JA, Carlson DS. The effects of pain from the mandibular joint and muscles on masticatory behavior in man. Arch Oral Biol 1988;33:175–182.

36. Glickman I, Carranza FA. Glickman's Clinical Periodontology, ed 7. Philadelphia: Saunders, 1990.

37. Gatter RA. Pharmacotherapeutics in fibrositis. Am J Med 1986;81(suppl 3A):63–66.

38. Kawai Y, et al. Studies in vivo measurements of oxidative stress in experimentally induced arthritis of the TMJ. Bull Kanagawa Dent Coll 1993;32:136–139.

39. Kozeniauskas JJ, Ralph WJ. Bilateral arthrographic evaluation of unilateral temporomandibular joint pain and dysfunction. J Prosthet Dent 1988;60:98–105.

40. Kubota E, Suga M, Shimizu S, et al. Reactive arthritis of the temporomandibular joint. Bull Kanagawa Dent Coll 2004;32:49–51.

41. Kubota E, et al. Oxidative stress and temporomandibular joint dysfunction. Bull Kanagawa Dent Coll 2002;30:141–145.

42. Lamey PJ, Taylor JA, Devine J. Giant cell arteritis: A forgotten diagnosis? Br Dent J 1988;164(2): 48–49.

43. Mongini F, Schmid W. Craniomandibular and TMJ Orthopedics. Chicago: Quintessence, 1989.

44. Hall LT. Physical therapy treatment results for 178 patients with TMJ syndrome. Am J Otol 1984;5:183–196.

45. Faulkner MG, Hatcher DC, Hay A. A three-dimensional investigation of the temporomandibular joint loading. J Biomech 1987;20:997–1002.

46. Matteson SR, Bechtold W, Phillips C, Staab EV. A method for three-dimensional image reformation for quantitative cephalometric analysis. J Oral Maxillofac Surg 1989;47:1053–1061.

47. Scapino RP. The posterior attachment: Its structure, function, and appearance in TMJ imaging studies. 1. J Craniomandib Disord 1991;5:83–95.

48. Scapino RP. The posterior attachment: Its structure, function, and appearance in TMJ imaging studies. 2. J Craniomandib Disord 1991;5:155–166.

49. Rovit RL, Murali R, Janetta PJ. Trigeminal Neuralgia. Baltimore: Williams & Wilkins, 1990.

50. Bianchi AL, Grélot L, Miller AD, King GL (eds). Mechanisms and Control of Emesis. London: Libbey, 1992:51–58.

51. Gunzburg R, Szpalski M. Whiplash Injuries. Philadelphia: Lippincott-Raven, 1998.

52. dos Santos J Jr. Injúrias cervicais nos casos de colisões automotivas [webpage in Portuguese]. Available at: http://www.portugal-linha.pt/opiniao/Jsantos/cron2.html.

53. Kolbinson DA, Epstein JB, Senthilselvan A, Burgess JA. Effect of impact and injury characteristics on post-motor vehicle accident temporomandibular disorders. Oral Surg Oral Med Oral Pathol Oral Radiol Endod 1998;85:665–673.

54. Miller DB. Low velocity impact, vehicular damage and passenger injury. Cranio 1998;16:226–229.

55. Barsh LI. Providing therapy for snoring and sleep apnea starts with knowledge of key terms, tests, and limits of care. 1. Dent Prod Rep 1999;Feb.

56. Thornton WK. Should the dentist independently assess and treat sleep-disordered breathing? J Calif Dent Assoc 1998;26:599–608.

57. Hilloowala R, Trent RB, Gunel E, Pifer RG. Proposed cephalometric diagnosis for osteogenic obstructive sleep apnea (OSA): The mandible/pharyngeal ratio. Cranio 1999;17:280–288.

58. Smith SD. A three-dimensional airway assessment for the treatment of snoring and/or sleep apnea with jaw repositioning intraoral appliances: A case study. Cranio 1996;14:332–344.

59. Yamamoto I, et al. Changes in sleep disorders after operation of the ankyloglossia with deviation of the epiglottis and larynx. Bull Kanagawa Dent Coll 2005;33:106–108.

60. Bernstein AK, Reidy RM. The effects of mandibular repositioning on obstructive sleep apnea. Cranio 1988;6:179–181.

61. Bonham PE, Currier GF, Orr WC, Othman J, Nanda RS. The effect of a modified functional appliance on obstructive sleep apnea. Am J Orthod Dentofac Orthop 1988;94:384–392.

62. Raphaelson MA, Alpher EJ, Bakker KW, Perlstrom JR. Oral appliance therapy for obstructive sleep apnea syndrome: Progressive mandibular advancement during polysomnography. Cranio 1998;16:44–50.

63. Schmidt-Nowara WW, Meade TE, Hays MB. Treatment of snoring and obstructive sleep apnea with a dental orthosis. Chest 1991;99:1378–1385.

DIAGNOSIS AND TREATMENT PROTOCOL

It is often challenging for the clinician to diagnose and treat a patient who has occlusal problems, temporomandibular disorders, and/or facial pain. The clinician must employ a sound clinical protocol for evaluating and managing patients with these conditions. A logical, effective protocol is described in this chapter.

PATIENT INTERVIEW

The first consultation, or interview, between the clinician and the patient often suggests that something formal is going to occur. However, this is not necessarily true. During the first interview with the patient, the clinician assesses the patient's feelings, fears, and expectations about the dental problem and asks why the patient believes that treatment is necessary. A patient's problems may range from simple conditions to a complex variety of signs, symptoms, and emotions. Sometimes, deeper, pertinent questioning will reveal the cause of the patient's problem or at least an indirect link with it. In addition, other interdisciplinary consultations might be useful to modify not only the course of the therapy but also the outcome and prognosis of the prescribed treatment.

During the initial interview, it is helpful to let the patient present the analysis of his or her problem. This may reveal the chronicity of possible problems and corresponding signs and symptoms as well as provide a progressive overview of features that may identify the stages of the disease or dysfunctional process. The well-conducted interview will very likely reveal the patient's attitude toward the condition and treatment. This aids the clinician's rational expectation of how much success may be achieved in solving the patient's clinical problem.

PATIENT EVALUATION

Once the interview with the patient is finished, it is time to start the diagnostic process. It is first necessary to assess whether the patient exhibits the most relevant normal occlusal functions of the masticatory system:

- Opening and closing mandibular movements without restrictions or limitations
- Gliding eccentric functional movements between the maxilla and mandible without interferences, especially on the balancing side
- Bilateral distribution of the masticatory force on a large number of teeth in intercuspal position of the maxilla and mandible (Fig 4-1)
- Axial loading of the teeth, producing minimal formation of horizontal components of force (see Fig 4-1)
- Acceptable interocclusal distance

If dysfunction is suspected, it is helpful to consistently evaluate these cardinal categories of symptoms, mnemonically represented by the expression *PSALM*:

- P: Pain
- S: Sounds from the joints, such as clicking or crepitus
- A: Alterations (incoordination) of mandibular movements
- L: Limitation of mandibular movements
- M: Muscular tenderness, fatigue, weakness, etc

During the evaluation process it is very difficult to separate one step from the other, because one symptom may prevail over others, or symptoms may even combine. This sequence of steps does not indicate any chronology or order of importance. The only relevant aspect is to avoid missing some step of the diagnostic sequence. For example, pain may be reported by the patient during assessment of another symptom, and the evaluation of joint noises may require more specific diagnostic methods throughout the phases of the examination process.

Pain

In the overall sequence of evaluation, pain may be considered a relevant symptom.[1] Pain is a great motivator. Patients most often seek treatment because they hurt. There is nothing in life more disturbing to human nature than pain. During the evaluation of pain, the clinician should assess its onset, intensity, quality, duration, localization, behavior, and so on. However, pain should be analyzed judiciously, because it may

Fig 4-1 Occlusal relationships along the long axis of opposing molars under the action of the masticatory force. A stable occlusal relationship may be achieved when the masticatory force is simultaneously directed to all quadrants of the opposing dental arches, analogous to what occurs in a force polygon, as represented by a four-legged stool.

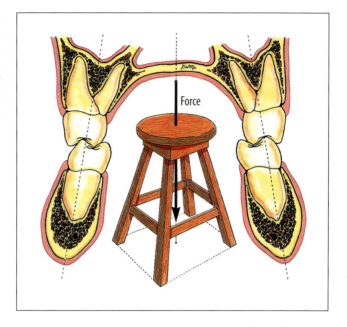

be misleading because of its subjective nature and the probability that some discomfort may be produced during the clinical examination. One of the most significant aspects of pain evaluation is the assessment of its chronicity and, accordingly, the need for immediate treatment (as in cases of acute pain).

A differential diagnosis of the sources of pain, especially in patients with temporomandibular disorders, may require evaluation and treatment of the patient by other medical specialists, such as an otolaryngologist or a neurologist. Some of these related painful entities may include migraine headaches, trigeminal neuralgia, ear disorders, angiomas, and brain tumors.

Joint sounds

The presence and nature of joint noises[2] can be confirmed with bilateral digital palpation. The clinician inserts the little finger of each hand in the external auditory meatus of the patient, and with gentle forward pressure, tries to feel the posterior surface of the condylar head. The patient is instructed or cued to move his or her mandible into protrusion, lateral movements, and wide open position. Any abnormal or grating movement of the condyles can be felt with this approach. However, a stethoscope can better define the characteristics of the noises that may be present (clicking or crepitus), as well as the clashing sound of premature contact of opposing dental cusps during mandibular closure.

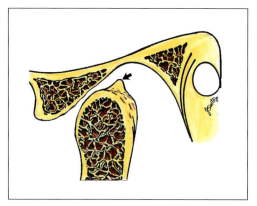

Fig 4-2 Altered TMJ with erosion of the articular eminence, resorption of the anterior portion of the condyle, and spur formation *(arrow)* on the upper pole of the condyle.

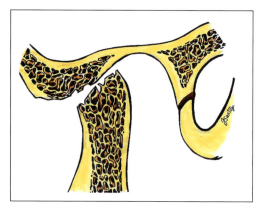

Fig 4-3 Rupture of compact bone continuity in both the upper pole of the condyle and articular eminence.

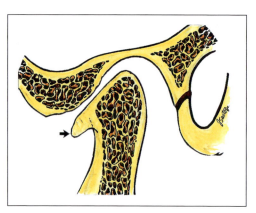

Fig 4-4 Condylar degeneration and osteophyte formation *(arrow)*.

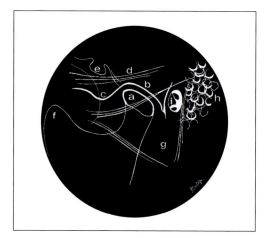

Fig 4-5 Simplified diagram of a transcranial radiograph of the TMJ. (a) Head of the condyle; (b) roof of the glenoid fossa, in relation to the base of the skull; (c) articular eminence; (d) base of the skull; (e) sella turcica; (f) coronoid process; (g) limits of the petrous portion of the temporal bone; (h) air cells of the mastoid process; (i) auditory meatus.

The selection of the different types of radiographs[3,4] must be based on the clinician's suspicion of the severity of the temporomandibular joint (TMJ) internal derangement (Figs 4-2 to 4-4). In the majority of cases, the clinician can start with transcranial or transfacial radiographs (Fig 4-5). If the patient is thought to have a deranged disc, an arthrogram may be indicated (Figs 4-6 to 4-9). However, if diagnostic confirmation is needed to assess more complex cases, diagnostic studies may be indicated including, among others, TMJ tomograms, computed tomography, and magnetic resonance images.[5]

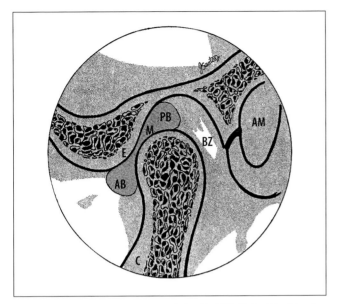

Fig 4-6 Arthrographic representation of a healthy TMJ. (C) Condyle; (E) articular eminence; (AB) anterior band of the disc; (M) articular disc; (PB) posterior band of the disk; (BZ) bilaminar zone; (AM) auditory meatus.

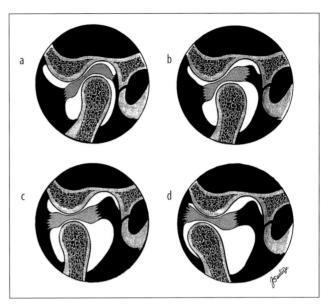

Fig 4-7 Diagram of normal TMJ arthrograms. The sequence shows the dispersion of the radiographic contrast in the lower and upper joint spaces of the TMJ during movements of the condyle, starting from maximum intercuspation *(a)*; the beginning of jaw opening *(b)*; half distance on opening *(c)*; and maximum opening *(d)*.

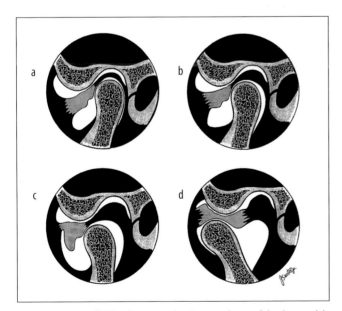

Fig 4-8 Diagram of TMJ arthrograms showing asynchrony of the disc-condyle complex. *(a)* Maximum intercuspation; *(b)* the beginning of jaw opening; *(c)* half opening; *(d)* maximum opening.

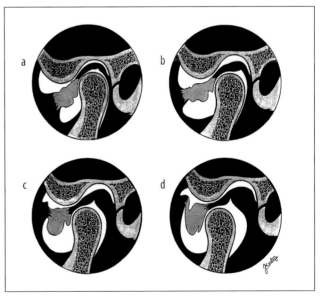

Fig 4-9 Diagram of TMJ arthrograms showing an open lock (disc displacement). *(a)* Maximum intercuspation; *(b)* the beginning of jaw opening; *(c)*, half opening; *(d)* maximum opening.

Alterations of mandibular motion

To evaluate the degree of coordination of mandibular movements, the patient is asked to move the mandible in several different directions, starting from centric position. Likewise, it is helpful to determine the degree of precision and comfort the patient has while returning back to the original centric position. During this stage of the diagnostic evaluation, it is appropriate to relate the findings to the levels of the dentition and occlusion. For example, during this assessment, it is possible to detect the incoordination of mandibular movements associated with gross occlusal interferences. Other correlated findings are inadequate molar support, excessive centric slides, a malocclusion (which produces instability of dental arches), and subtle occlusal interferences. All of these are very likely to be the response of the neuromuscular system to hold the mandible in a comfortable position.[6]

Eventually, the best way to clinically test mandibular incoordination is to ask the patient to snap the jaws shut sharply, to ascertain that the teeth are tapping together. Bilateral occlusal contacts should occur simultaneously and produce a characteristic knocking sound.

Limitations of mandibular movements

Temporomandibular disorders include internal derangements, chronic and acute traumatic arthritis, osteoarthritis, progressive degeneration of the joints, congenital deformities, and other problems. All these entities are capable of limiting and modifying the pattern of mandibular motion (Fig 4-10). The mandibular range of movement must be checked in all directions of mandibular displacement.

Patterns of limited mandibular movements are diagnostic clues about TMJ disorders. For instance, if the limitation of the mandibular movement subsides after the joint pops and the noise is accompanied by deviation toward the affected side, the clinician may suspect an internal derangement of the disc (anterior dislocation of the disc with reduction; see Fig 4-10), which may accompany other clicking sounds.

Another typical TMJ disorder is associated with severe restriction of mouth opening (25 mm or less) with slight deviation of the mandible to one side (Fig 4-11). There may be grating noises inside the temporomandibular joints. In this case, the clinician may suspect anterior disc derangement without reduction, accompanied by osteoarthritic degeneration of the articular surfaces.

If the limitation occurs mutually with acute muscular spasm in the absence or presence of a clicking sound, it may be due to muscle trismus. In this case, an acute muscular disorder (such as irritation of the muscles following the removal of a third molar) may be responsible for the problem. For example, spasm of the

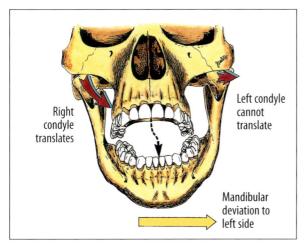

Fig 4-10 Left deviation of the mandible *(yellow and black arrows)* during opening, probably caused by a functional problem inside the joint *(red arrows)*.

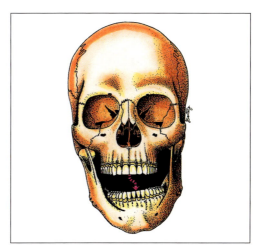

Fig 4-11 Typical example of limited opening with deviation of the mandible to one side *(arrow)*.

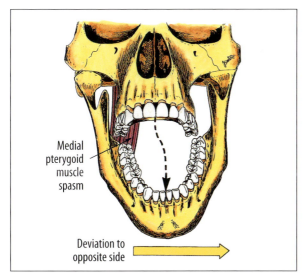

Fig 4-12 Left-side deviation of the mandible *(yellow and black arrows)* during opening as a result of spasm of the right medial pterygoid muscle.

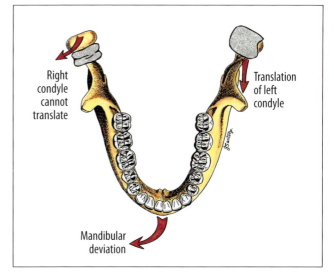

Fig 4-13 Mandible with a tendency to deviate to the right side during protrusive movement because of anterior displacement of the disc within the right joint.

medial pterygoid muscle on the right side may cause the mandible to deviate to the opposite side on opening (Fig 4-12).

Severely limited lateral and protrusive movements could also suggest ankylosis of the temporomandibular joints. If there is an anterior displacement of the disc in one of the joints, the affected joint cannot allow proper translation of the condyle during protrusive movement. In this case, if the disc is displaced in the right TMJ or if there is ankylosis of the right TMJ, the mandible will deviate to the right side during protrusive movement (Fig 4-13).

Masticatory muscles

The masticatory muscles should be evaluated with a consistent sequence of bilateral (whenever possible) digital palpation techniques to assess the presence of dysfunctional symptoms or discomfort. It is always necessary to be gentle with the patient to avoid initiating discomfort and false results. Muscle palpation has relative value in the diagnosis of temporomandibular disorders, because the primary source of pain may occur in another area of the body and be referred to a masticatory muscle. Nevertheless, it is possible that during palpation the clinician may come across trigger points in the muscle.[7] These trigger points are painful areas with very low threshold for direct stimulation; ie, a gentle touch will cause severe pain.

DIAGNOSTIC PALPATION

The method of palpation should be uniform and consistent for all patients. Therefore, the clinician should start and finish the sequence with the patient's head in equivalent positions, to avoid the risk of missing an area. It is a good idea to always start with extraoral palpation and then proceed to intraoral regions.

Extraoral palpation

Temporomandibular joint

The temporomandibular joints are palpated first to check for sounds, movements, and pain (Fig 4-14). The lateral areas of the joints can be palpated bilaterally in the preauricular area, immediately in front of the ear tragus (Fig 4-15). The clinician can palpate the area behind the condyles by inserting his or her little finger in the patient's external meatus. All findings during this procedure should be recorded in the patient's chart.

Deep layer of the masseter muscle

The second area to be checked is the deep portion of the masseter muscle. Using the middle and index fingers of each hand, the clinician produces gentle, simultaneous bilateral pressure on each side of the patient's face. The area palpated is the shallow

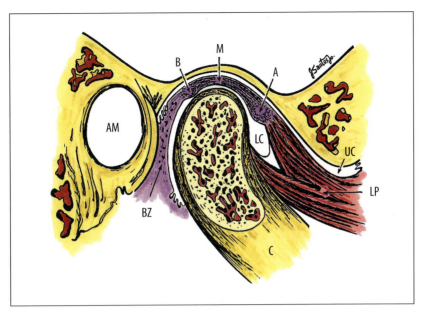

Fig 4-14 Anatomic structures of the temporomandibular joint. (M) Meniscus; (C) condyle; (AM) auditory meatus; (LP) lateral pterygoid muscle; (A) anterior band; (B) posterior band; (BZ), bilaminar zone; (LC) lower compartment; (UC) upper compartment.

depression of the skin at the level of the sigmoid notch of the mandible (see Fig 4-15). The group of fibers of this portion of the muscle is primarily in charge of the retrusive range of mandibular movements and frequently becomes sensitive during episodes of bruxism, especially when bruxism is associated with deflective occlusal contacts in centric relation.

Anterior border and body of the masseter muscle

The superficial portion of the masseter muscle overlays a large part of the deep layer. This portion of the muscle has a long, tendinous attachment to the zygomatic arch, and the bulk of its muscular structure nears the mandibular angle. During simultaneous bilateral palpation (see Fig 4-15), the clinician checks for painful areas, as well as for the sequence of contraction when the patient squeezes the teeth together. As a powerful mandibular elevator muscle (Fig 4-16), the masseter often becomes sensitive during aggressive bruxism habits and TMJ problems. Even the palpation of the anterior border of this muscle can disclose important diagnostic information (see Fig 4-15).

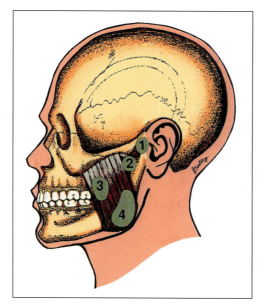

Fig 4-15 Extraoral palpation sequence. (1) Temporomandibular joint area; (2) deep layer of the masseter muscle; (3) anterior border of the superficial layer of the masseter muscle; (4) body of the masseter muscle.

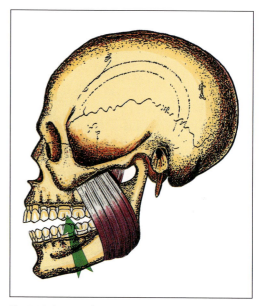

Fig 4-16 Anatomic location and action *(arrow)* of the masseter muscle.

Temporalis muscle

The fan-shaped fibers of this muscle that attach to the sides of the skull are defined in different functional areas. The anterior and intermediate bundles of this muscle are partially responsible for mandibular elevation and very sensitive to some occlusal interferences (Fig 4-17). The posterior bundle, because of its horizontal and backward orientation, produces retrusive action during mandibular movements (Fig 4-18). These bundles can be palpated extraorally for symptoms and contraction patterns (Fig 4-19).

Medial pterygoid muscle

This muscle, internally located in relation to the ascending ramus of the mandible, runs almost parallel to the masseter muscle. During mandibular elevation, both muscles have a combined function (synergistic action). However, the medial pterygoid muscle also assists in lateral excursions of the mandible (Fig 4-20). The best way to palpate this muscle extraorally is to assess the area of its insertion on the internal medial surface of the lower border of the mandible (Fig 4-21). Because a large part of the body of this muscle is located inside the mouth, intraoral palpation is totally hindered by other anatomic structures.

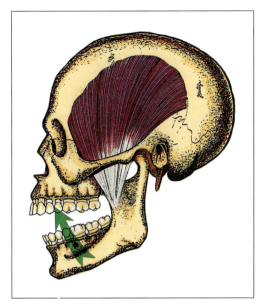

Fig 4-17 Anatomic location and action *(arrow)* of the temporalis muscle.

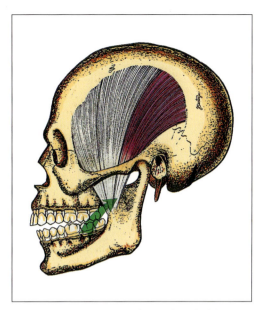

Fig 4-18 Anatomic location and action *(arrow)* of the posterior band of the temporalis muscle.

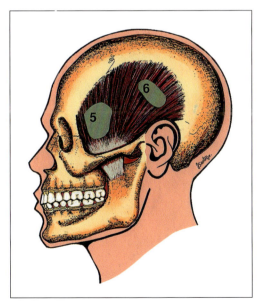

Fig 4-19 Extraoral palpation sequence. (5) Anterior and middle bands of the temporalis muscle; (6) posterior band of the temporalis muscle.

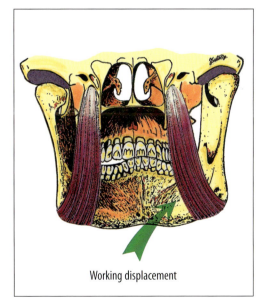

Fig 4-20 Anatomic location and right-side muscle contraction *(arrow)* of the medial pterygoid muscle.

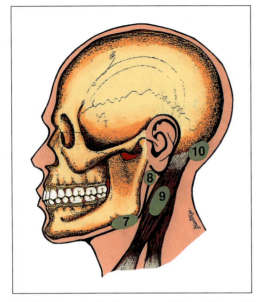

Fig 4-21 Extraoral palpation sequence. (7) Area of the medial pterygoid muscle insertion, at the level of the mandibular gonial process; (8) area of the posterior belly of the digastric muscle; (9) body of the sternocleidomastoid muscle; (10) insertion of muscles in the occipital area.

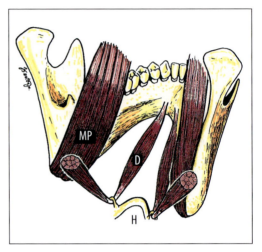

Fig 4-22 Suprahyoid musculature in the mandible. (MP) Medial pterygoid muscle; (D) digastric muscle; (H) hyoid bone.

Posterior belly of the digastric muscle

The digastric muscle, an important depressor of the mandible (Fig 4-22), may be sensitive to some forms of TMJ dysfunction. The clinician should palpate this muscle with gentle digital pressure below the angle of the mandible (see Fig 4-21).

Head and cervical musculature

If the clinician suspects that the patient is experiencing referred pain, or if the patient is complaining of a problem related to posture, the clinician should palpate the muscles of the head and neck, although these muscles are not necessarily involved in the masticatory process. In general, palpation of the sternocleidomastoid (see Fig 4-21), occipital (see Fig 4-21), and trapezius muscles (Fig 4-23) may reveal important diagnostic information.

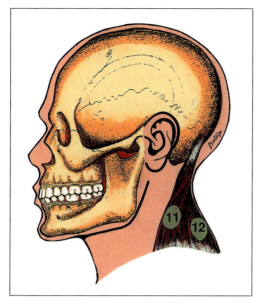

Fig 4-23 Extraoral palpation sequence. (11 and 12) Portions of the trapezius muscle.

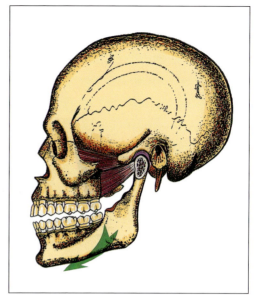

Fig 4-24 Anatomic location and action *(arrow)* of the lateral pterygoid muscle.

Intraoral palpation

The following sequence of palpation is accomplished with unilateral palpation. The oral mucosa is very sensitive, and care must be taken to avoid false results of pain. The clinician must be very gentle during this phase of the evaluation.

Insertion of the temporalis muscle

The temporalis muscle has its tendinous insertion on the coronoid process and anterior border of the mandibular ramus (see Figs 4-17 and 4-18). Hence, this anatomic region should be palpated internally. In general, as a positioner of the mandible, this muscle is sensitive to occlusal discrepancies, especially those related to centric and eccentric mandibular positions.

Lateral pterygoid muscle

The palpation of this area may involve assessments of muscles other than the lateral pterygoid muscle (Fig 4-24). Some authors have referred to this as *palpation of the pterygoid window*. Others state that the lateral pterygoid muscle cannot be palpated because it resides too deeply in relation to many anatomic structures.

107

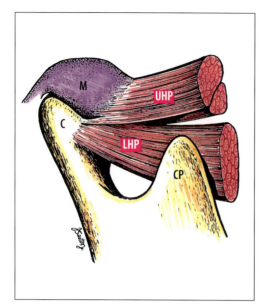 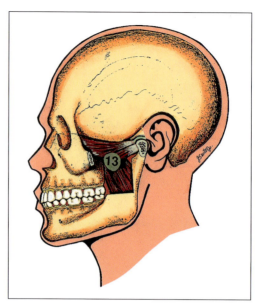

Fig 4-25 Anatomic relationships of the lateral pterygoid muscle to the structures of the TMJ. (M) Meniscus; (UHP) upper head of the muscle; (LHP) lower head of the muscle; (C) condyle; (CP) coronoid process.

Fig 4-26 Intraoral palpation sequence. (13) Pterygoid window behind the maxillary tuberosity.

It is difficult to predict if this type of palpation will reach all areas of the lateral pterygoid muscle (superior, intermediate, and inferior heads), because anatomically the inferior head is the nearest to this area (Fig 4-25).

The location of the pterygoid window is represented by a narrow access behind the maxillary tuberosity, in an upward direction. The palpation is done unilaterally using the little finger with very gentle pressure (Fig 4-26). Factors that limit mandibular movements—occlusal prematurities in centric position and eccentric interferences—may produce increased sensitivity of this group of muscles.

PROVOCATIVE TEST

In maximum intercuspation, the condyles are subject to small magnitudes of masticatory force while, at the same time, they should assume a stable position in their respective glenoid fossa. However, if a separator is interposed between molars (eg, a cotton roll, tongue depressor, or wooden blade), there is a tendency for different reactions because masticatory forces produce axial displacement of the condyles in the joints. Therefore, having the patient occlude on a separator,

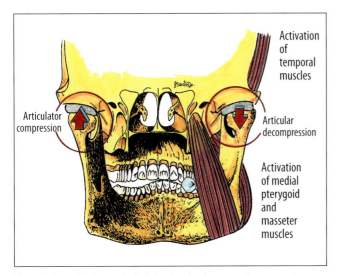

Fig 4-27 Posterior view of the skull showing the placement of a separator between right molars for a right-side provocative test.

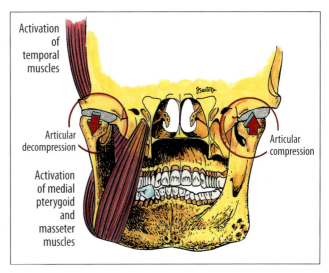

Fig 4-28 Posterior view of the skull showing the placement of the separator between left molars for a left-side provocative test.

for no more than 60 seconds, may constitute a valuable complementary diagnostic tool to check for the presence of temporomandibular joint and masticatory pains.

If the patient is asked to bite on a cotton roll or tongue depressor, different forces will be produced in the joints, depending on the side in which the separator is interposed. When occluding on the separator, the patient is apt to produce decreased pressure in the joint of the same side of the head (ipsilateral side) and increased pressure on the other side (contralateral side), resulting in increased activation of the temporalis, masseter, and medial pterygoid muscles on the same side of the head (Figs 4-27 and 4-28). This interplay between increase and decrease of pressure often reveals important clues related to temporomandibular joint symptoms. For example, if the increase of pressure in the joint elicits or increases pain, the interpretation is that there is indeed some disorder within the articular structures. If decreased pressure in the joint elicits or increases pain, the problem is probably related to extracapsular structures and may even involve masticatory muscles. If the separator is placed between the incisors, pressure in both joints will be increased simultaneously (Fig 4-29).

Other provocative tests can be instituted during the diagnostic evaluation, such as matching opposing atypical facets of wear on the dentition and asking the patient to occlude in this position for no more than 1 minute. This procedure may disclose masticatory muscle symptoms in patients with dysfunction.

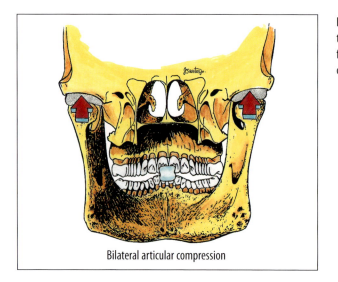

Fig 4-29 Posterior view of the skull showing the placement of a separator between incisors for an anterior provocative test in which articular compression occurs bilaterally *(arrows)*.

Bilateral articular compression

RESISTANCE TEST

To define the symptoms of some selected masticatory muscles during clinical examination, the clinician may exert controlled resistance tests on the patient's mandible using manual pressure. These tests may involve the following protocol:

1. To detect the symptomatic response of the lateral pterygoid muscles, protrusion against resistance (Fig 4-30) may activate these muscles on both sides of the head.
2. To detect pain response in the right lateral and medial pterygoid muscles, resistance against left lateral movement may be exerted on the side of the mandible (Fig 4-31). Resistance against right lateral movement (Fig 4-32) may provide reciprocal response of the left lateral and medial pterygoid muscles.
3. Resistance against opening (Fig 4-33) will test for symptoms of the lateral pterygoid muscles.

OCCLUSAL RELATIONSHIPS

Occlusal contacts may be detected directly in the patient's mouth during different mandibular relationships. In addition, the use of mounted casts on semiadjustable articulators is a well-accepted means to check for occlusal contacts and maxillo-mandibular relationships.

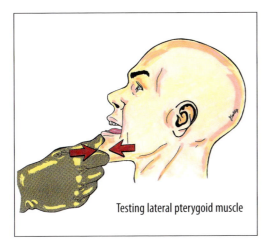

Testing lateral pterygoid muscle

Fig 4-30 Resistance test when pressure *(arrows)* is exerted to counteract protrusive movement of the mandible.

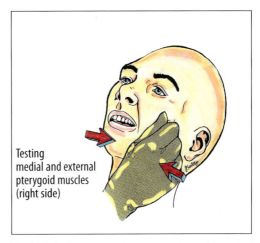

Testing medial and external pterygoid muscles (right side)

Fig 4-31 Resistance test when pressure *(arrows)* is exerted on the left side of the face to prevent left-side movement.

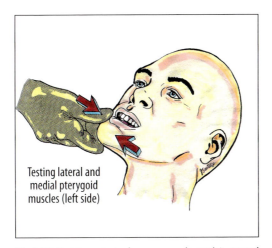

Testing lateral and medial pterygoid muscles (left side)

Fig 4-32 Resistance test when pressure *(arrows)* is exerted on the right side of the face to hinder right lateral movement of the mandible.

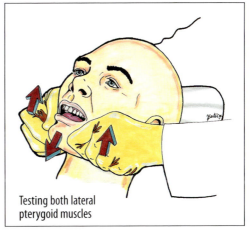

Testing both lateral pterygoid muscles

Fig 4-33 Resistance test when pressure *(arrows)* is exerted to prevent jaw opening.

Some clinical aspects of the functional analysis of occlusion are related to the influence of some distorted interocclusal relationships and the instability of the masticatory system. The absence of teeth, the degree of tooth mobility, the presence of atypical facets of wear, tooth sensitivity, crown fractures, root fractures, trauma from occlusion, and other findings, are all prominent factors that must be considered while the treatment plan is prepared.

The most probable immediate outcome of any comprehensive occlusal analysis will be the indication for an occlusal adjustment.

DIAGNOSTIC TOOLS

Several diagnostic tools are available to the dental profession.[5,8–19] Yearly, new and more sophisticated equipment becomes available. What should be understood is that diagnostic tests using instruments should be done only when it is absolutely necessary. In most cases, the use of sophisticated equipment is not worth the time, money, and effort spent, if an accurate diagnosis can be obtained with just simple approaches. In addition, information obtained through the use of any type of instrument should be used as only part of diagnostic data and not as a sole factor on which to base a diagnosis. No equipment is absolutely reliable. If instruments are used, then the operator should be completely sure that he or she is able to deliver the correct interpretation of the results obtained from the tests.

The diagnosis of complex cases never should be based on a single diagnostic tool. Rather, it should be based on the composite results obtained from various diagnostic tools and the use of mounted diagnostic casts on the articulator.

TREATMENT PLANNING

The most rational approach to treatment planning is for the clinician to use his or her best judgment, based on thorough clinical evaluation, to achieve a preliminary diagnosis and to establish a treatment plan that is essentially conservative. Depending on the patient's response to the initial phase of treatment, a more definitive diagnosis can then be made, bringing with it a more reliable prognosis for the clinical solution. Thus, in the patient's interest, the initial therapy should be based on management of symptoms with conservative methods, such as physiotherapy, behavior modification through counseling and dietary restriction, mild medications, and the institution of occlusal splint therapy (this approach in some cases may act more as a diagnostic tool than a treatment appliance).[20–26]

It is important to emphasize that initial therapy should be reversible, because it is correlated to the amount of information that must be gathered during the process of reaching the final diagnosis and prognosis. In more advanced stages of the treatment process, irreversible types of therapy, such as occlusal adjustment, oral reconstruction, orthodontics, and orthognathic surgery, may be indicated.

REFERENCES

1. Akil H, Lewis JW (eds). Neurotransmitters and Pain Control. Vol 9: Pain and headache. Basel: Karger, 1987.

2. Barghi N, dos Santos J Jr, Narendran S. Effects of posterior teeth replacement on temporomandibular joint sounds. J Prosthet Dent 1992;69:132–136.

3. Scapino RP. The posterior attachment: Its structure, function, and appearance in TMJ imaging studies. 1. J Craniomandib Disord 1991;5:83–95.

4. Scapino RP. The posterior attachment: Its structure, function, and appearance in TMJ imaging studies. 2. J Craniomandib Disord 1991;5:155–166.

5. Schellhas KP, Fritts HM, Heithoff KB, Jahn JA, Wilkes CH, Omlie MR. Temporomandibular joint: MR fast scanning. Cranio 1988;6:209–216.

6. McCarthy WL Jr, Darnell MW. Rehabilitation of the temporomandibular joint through the application of motion. Cranio 1993;11:298–307.

7. Jaeger B, Reeves JL. Quantification of changes in myofascial trigger point sensitivity with pressures algometer following passive stretch. Pain 1986;27:203–210.

8. Conti PCR. Low level laser therapy in the treatment of temporomandibular disorders (TMD): A double blind pilot study. Cranio 1997;15:144–149.

9. Cooper BC. The role of bioelectronic instruments in documenting and managing temporomandibular disorders. J Am Dent Assoc 1996;127:1611–1614.

10. dos Santos J Jr, Giordani AI. Estimulaciones con frecuencias altas y bajas mezcladas en el tratamiento de las alteraciones temporomandibulares. Mediante la utilización del nuevo instrumiento "TENS." J Clin Odontol 1994/1995;10(3):63–68.

11. Ersek RA. Pain Control with Transcutaneous Electrical Neurostimulation. St Louis: Green, 1981.

12. Jankelson B, Sparks S, Crane PF, Radke JC. Neural conduction of the myo-monitor stimulus. A quantitative analysis. J Prosthet Dent 1975;34:245–253.

13. Jankelson B, Radke JC. The myo-monitor: Its use and abuse. Quintessence Int 1978;9(2):47–52.

14. Lark MR, Gangarosa LP. Iontophoresis: An effective modality for the treatment of inflammatory disorders of the temporomandibular joint and myofascial pain. Cranio 1990;8:108–119.

15. Mohl ND, Ohrbach RK, Crow HC, Gross AJ. Devices for the diagnosis and treatment of temporomandibular disorders. 3. Thermography, ultrasound, electrical stimulation and electromyographic biofeedback. J Prosthet Dent 1990;63:472–477.

16. Nelson SJ, dos Santos J Jr, Barghi N, Narendran S. Using moist heat to treat acute temporomandibular muscle pain dysfunction. Compend Contin Educ Dent 1991;12:808–816.

17. Nelson SJ, Ash MM. An evaluation of a moist heating pad for the treatment of TMJ/muscle pain dysfunction. Cranio 1988;6:355–359.

18. Wessberg GA, Carroll WL, Dinham R, Wolford LM. Transcutaneous electrical stimulation as an adjunct in the management of myofascial pain dysfunction syndrome. J Prosthet Dent 1981;45:307–314.

19. Zwijnenburg AJ, Kroon GW, Verbeeten B Jr, Naeije M. Jaw movement responses to electrical stimulation of different parts of the human temporalis muscle. J Dent Res 1996;75:1798–1803.

20. dos Santos J Jr, de Rijk W. Vectorial analysis of the equilibrium of forces transmitted to TMJ and occlusal bite plane splints. J Oral Rehabil 1995;22:301–310.

21. dos Santos J Jr, Nowlin TP. The effect of splint therapy on TMJ position measured by the Gerber Resiliency Test. J Oral Rehabil 1992;19:663–670.

22. Humsi ANK, Naeije M, Hippe JA, Hansson TL. The immediate effects of a stabilization splint on the muscular symmetry in the masseter and anterior temporal muscles of patients with a craniomandibular disorder. J Prosthet Dent 1989;62:339–343.

23. Okeson JP. Long-term treatment of disk-interference disorders of the temporomandibular joint with anterior repositioning occlusal splints. J Prosthet Dent 1988;60:611–616.

24. Shi CS, Wang HY. Postural and maximum activity in elevators during mandible pre- and post-occlusal splint treatment of temporomandibular joint disturbance syndrome. J Oral Rehabil. 1989;16:155–161.

25. Suvinen T, Reade P. Prognostic features of value in the management of temporomandibular joint pain dysfunction syndrome by occlusal splint therapy. J Prosthet Dent 1989;61:355–361.

26. Turk DC, Zaki HS, Rudy TE. Effects of intraoral appliance and biofeedback/stress management alone and in combination in treating pain and depression in patients with temporomandibular disorders. J Prosthet Dent 1993;70:158–164.

FABRICATION OF OCCLUSAL BITE SPLINTS

This chapter presents the use of heat-cured and self-cured acrylic for the fabrication of occlusal bite splints. The heat-cured acrylic is indicated for laboratory use, while the self-cured acrylic can be used chairside when required for urgent patient care. Both appliances have the same morphologic configuration.

LABORATORY FABRICATION

This section will describe the fabrication of a clear, heat-cured acrylic resin occlusal bite plane splint that will be processed in the laboratory. Although there are numerous designs of occlusal splints, the model described in this section is a maxillary splint. It has the following characteristics: all the maxillary teeth are covered; the external mandibular surface must be smooth for mandibular tooth contact; and the splint must have bilateral anterior canine guidance (Fig 5-1).

Use of an articulator

Bite splints may be fabricated using semiadjustable articulators. (For mounting procedures refer to chapter 2.) Figure 5-2 shows an example of mounting casts on a hypothetical articulator and relating the mandibular arch in maximum intercuspation (centric occlusion). The baseline settings of the instrument used in this example represent the usual adjustment for the majority of semiadjustable instruments.

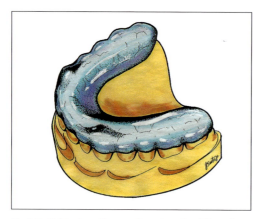

Fig 5-1 Finished maxillary acrylic resin occlusal bite splint.

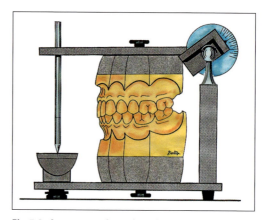

Fig 5-2 Casts mounted on a hypothetical arcon-type semi-adjustable articulator.

Initial settings

The articulator must be adjusted to a proper baseline setting. Over time, adjustable components of the articulator may inadvertently unfasten or may be intentionally modified according to other demands. The articulator should be set to its original settings before the casts are mounted.

Articulator adjustments

Taking into consideration the biomechanical specifications for the occlusal bite plane splint, the appliance must have anterior guidance for eccentric mandibular movements. For such, the incisal pin and incisal table must be set to disclude the posterior teeth. To obtain this setting, the clearance between opposing teeth must be checked when the instrument is guided in protrusive and lateral excursions. First, the anteroposterior inclination of the incisal table is adjusted (Fig 5-3) and then the angle of its lateral wings. The lateral wings are adjusted by moving the articulator laterally to one side and lifting the corresponding wing until it touches the incisal pin. The best setting is achieved when opposing canines are placed end to end (Fig 5-4). If the adjusted guidance is insufficient to clear the interference (or is too abrupt) it can be readjusted later, during waxup of the splint.

The thickness of the occlusal bite plane splint will be determined by extending the incisal pin. This produces the necessary interocclusal clearance for fabrication of the appliance. The splint thickness (vertical dimension) is estimated by verifying whether the occlusal plane of the maxillary arch clears the tips of the mandibular molar cusps at the most distal portion of the arches (Fig 5-5). The resulting clearance between opposing occlusal surfaces of the casts will provide room for the thickness of the acrylic resin. A practical way to define this clearance

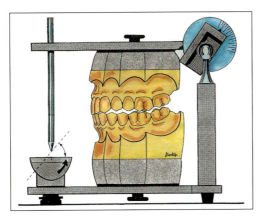

Fig 5-3 Setting the incisal table for protrusive movement *(arrows)*.

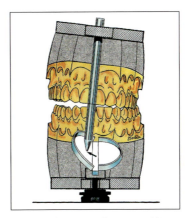

Fig 5-4 Adjustment of anterior guidance. *(arrow)* The lateral wings of the incisal table are elevated to comply with eccentric lateral movements.

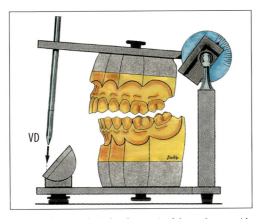

Fig 5-5 The incisal pin has been raised *(arrow)* to provide opposing tooth clearance for the fabrication of occlusal splint. (VD) Vertical dimension of the appliance.

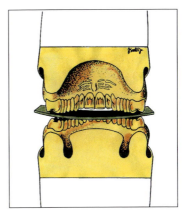

Fig 5-6 Insertion of a flexible plastic ruler or card between casts to adjust the length of the incisal pin.

is to insert a flexible plastic ruler or card between casts and adjust the length of the incisal pin (Fig 5-6).

In general, this vertical opening will provide a thickness of 2 mm of acrylic resin between occlusal surfaces (Fig 5-7). The thicker the appliance, the more the condyles will be displaced from their respective fossae (Figs 5-8 to 5-10). However, the splint thickness is determined by the nature of the interocclusal relationship (eg, the type of intercuspation, deep anterior overbite, anterior overjet, or tipped teeth). A common error is to insufficiently open the vertical dimension, which positions the mandibular buccal cusps very close together or even in contact and may result in perforation of the acrylic resin during adjustment of the appliance and balancing interferences.

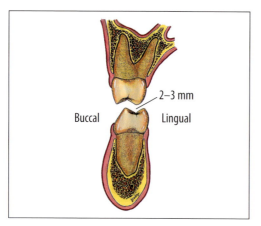

Fig 5-7 Usual distance (2 to 3 mm) between opposing occlusal surfaces to provide thickness to the appliance.

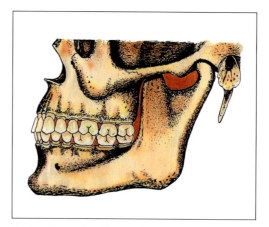

Fig 5-8 Relationship of the condyle to the joint in maximum intercuspation.

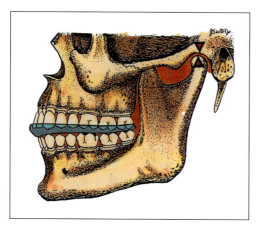

Fig 5-9 Relationship of the condyle to the joint *(red arrowheads)* when an occlusal splint with a moderate vertical dimension is inserted in the mouth.

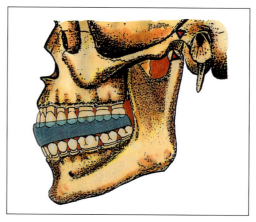

Fig 5-10 Anterior displacement of the condyle in the joint *(red arrowheads)* when a thick occlusal splint is inserted in the mouth.

Preparation of the casts

Once the articulator is set, the maxillary cast is prepared for splint construction. With a sharp-point pencil, the outline of the area to be covered by the appliance is drawn on the cast. The outline of the labial surfaces of the anterior teeth should extend just beyond the incisal edge, no more than 1 to 2 mm (Fig 5-11). This minimal amount of acrylic resin on the labial surface can provide some esthetics for the appliance, but its main purpose is to prevent jiggling of the anterior teeth.

The outline at the posterior area of the cast extends 2 to 3 mm onto the buccal surfaces. If the crowns of the teeth have a pronounced deviation toward the lingual

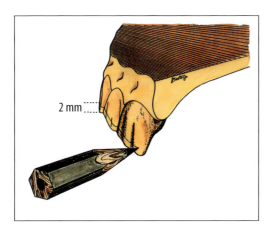

Fig 5-11 Outline of the buccal extension of the occlusal splint at the level of the maxillary anterior teeth. The extension should be limited to 1 to 2 mm cervically.

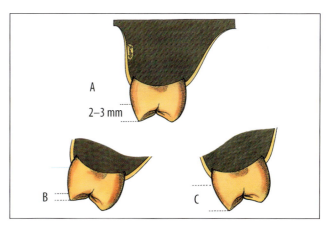

Fig 5-12 Variations in the buccal extension of the occlusal bite splint can be planned during the waxing of the appliance. (A) Average buccal extension in the presence of a normally upright molar; (B) reduced encroachment, because the long axis of the molar is tilted buccally; (C) greater encroachment of the extension on the height of contour of the crown of a maxillary molar, because its long axis is tilted lingually.

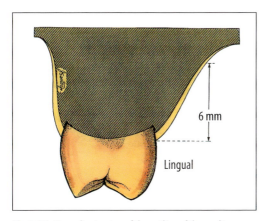

Fig 5-13 Lingual extension of the outline of the appliance.

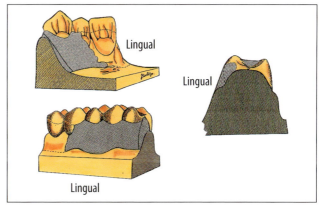

Fig 5-14 Blockout procedures. Areas of the cast are blocked out at the anterior and posterior teeth. The blockout is concentrated on the lingual side; for better retention of the appliance, no blockout is created on the buccal side.

area and the height of contour is close to the cervical line, then the outline must be extended 3 to 6 mm onto the buccal surfaces for extra retention (Fig 5-12).

The posterior extension of the appliance is just distal to the last tooth in the arch. The palatal outline extends 6 mm onto the attached gingiva, which will create a seal for retention and will increase the strength of the splint (Fig 5-13).

The cast is inspected to judge the path of insertion. To block out the undercuts of the cast on the lingual area, the cast is soaked and fast-setting plaster is added with a small brush (Fig 5-14). To enhance retention of the appliance, the buccal area is not blocked out.

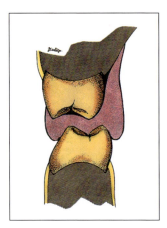

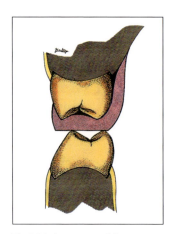

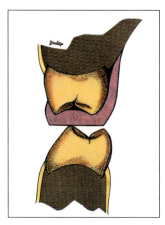

Fig 5-15 The first indentations are produced on the soft wax. The incisal pin must be touching the incisal table at this stage.

Fig 5-16 Appearance of the construction when excess wax is removed from the occlusal surface. Sometimes the size of the mandibular arch in relation to the maxillary arch produces a different contact relationship. It is necessary to create contact for both the buccal and lingual cusps if the occlusal surfaces are very wide.

Fig 5-17 Contact of the teeth in splint centric on the bite splint. If the mandibular posterior teeth are tipped lingually, only the buccal cusps are in contact with splint.

Waxup of the bite splint

Laboratory approaches

Softened regular pink baseplate wax is adapted to cover the outlined area. A warm waxing instrument is used to trim the excess and seal the margin of the wax to the cast. The articulator is closed and the incisal pin is brought into contact with the incisal table (Fig 5-15). If necessary, warm wax is added to promote contact for opposing teeth. All the incisal edges and buccal cusps must be included in the wax. The occlusal surface is shaved flat, but all the centric stops are retained. Articulating ribbon is used to visualize all centric stops (Figs 5-16 and 5-17). A flat occlusal surface will provide a smooth platform for new contact points as the patient's muscles relax and the mandible correspondingly adjusts to a more comfortable position. It also allows freedom during centric and Bennett movements (Fig 5-18).

Small portions of wax are attached at the canine areas for anterior guidance in lateral and protrusive excursions (Figs 5-19 to 5-25). In some cases, the protrusive guidance may be established for all anterior teeth. If there are any uncertainties about incorporating the incisors for guidance, the amount of the patient's overbite should be examined. It may be almost impossible to abolish contact on the incisors. In this circumstance, an anterior slope may be included to allow for light

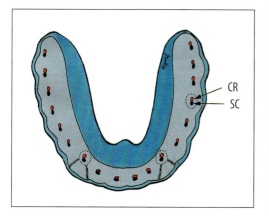

Fig 5-18 Occlusal aspect of the splint after all the contacts have been adjusted for splint centric (SC), centric relation (CR), and eccentric movements.

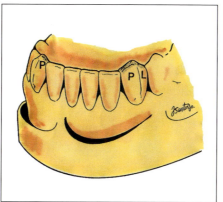

Fig 5-19 Areas of the mandibular canine cusps used for protrusive (P) and lateral (L) guidance, which are commonly used in the creation of anterior guidance in bite splints (left lateral view).

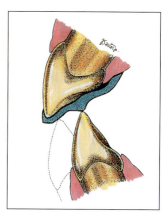

Fig 5-20 Canine guidance for protrusive movement. In cases of deep overbite, an anterior ramp often is used to provide protrusive guidance.

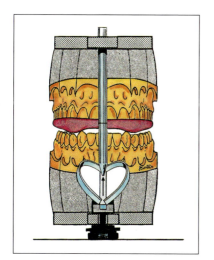

Fig 5-21 Adjustment of the incisal table *(arrow)* to provide protrusive guidance. The thickness of the wax and dimension of the guiding ramp of the future appliance was taken into consideration.

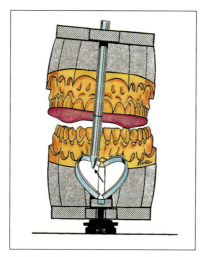

Fig 5-22 When the lateral wing of the occlusal table *(arrow)* is adjusted to accommodate lateral movement (in this example, left lateral movement), it is necessary to take into account the future thickness of the appliance and the dimension of the guiding ramp that will be waxed up.

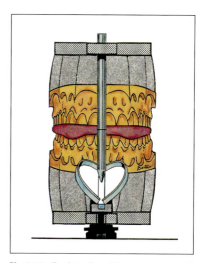

Fig 5-23 Checking the splint centric contact of the waxup.

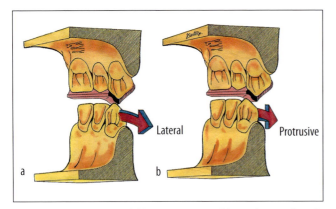

Fig 5-24 *(a)* Right lateral and *(b)* protrusive action of the guidance on the right side of an occlusal splint.

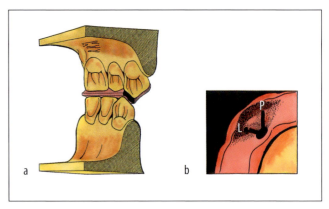

Fig 5-25 *(a)* Relationship of the mandibular canine to its guidance on the occlusal splint, in splint centric position. *(b)* Mandibular canine path in relation to its guidance during lateral (L) and protrusive (P) movements.

contact on the mandibular incisors (Fig 5-26). Enough wax should be added to eliminate all interferences, and nonfunctional areas should be reduced to improve esthetics and phonetics (especially *I* and *S* sounds).

The wax surface should be evened, and then the waxed splint should be inspected. After completion of the waxup, the amount of centric freedom on the occlusal surface of the splint should be confirmed, especially if the patient presents with a deep overbite and a small clearance between opposing molars (Fig 5-27). The canine guidance must present a controlled steepness without generating more than 1 to 2 mm clearance between the appliance and the posterior teeth of the opposing arch in working movement (Fig 5-28).

The tooth-supporting cusps should contact the splint during movement from centric relation to splint centric when there is proper canine guidance. *Splint centric* is considered that position where the patient bites on the appliance. The cusp tips of the mandibular canines should rest on the flat surface of the appliance before engaging in any protrusive or lateral guidance (Fig 5-29). This last requirement is relevant for comfort and compliance during the use of the occlusal splint.

Morphologic requirements of the splint

The wax covers 6 mm of attached gingiva on the lingual and occlusal surfaces and approximately 2 to 3 mm of the facial surfaces of maxillary teeth if the splint is fabricated on the maxillary arch (which in the majority of the cases is preferable for ease of construction and the patient's comfort) or mandibular teeth for mandibular appliances.

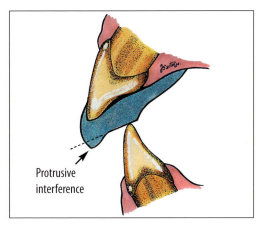

Fig 5-26 Relationship of the mandibular incisor to the contacting surface of the occlusal splint. *(dotted line)* Possible path of the incisors in protrusion and the excess contour that must be removed.

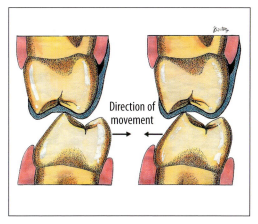

Fig 5-27 Lateral freedom for splints with a limited amount of vertical dimension opening.

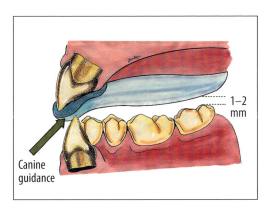

Fig 5-28 Proper anterior guidance of the occlusal splint must provide no more than 1- to 2-mm clearance between posterior teeth during working-side movement.

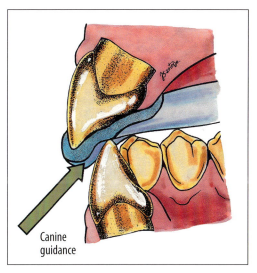

Fig 5-29 View of the occlusal splint at the level of the anterior guidance and the relationship between opposing canines. Note the flat area in front of the mandibular canine to provide freedom in centric.

The occlusal surface must be smooth, with occlusal contact in splint centric for all opposing teeth. The occluding surface must be perpendicular to the long axis of the opposing teeth to impart occlusal loads along the long axis of the teeth and thereby avoid unstable tipping forces (Fig 5-30).

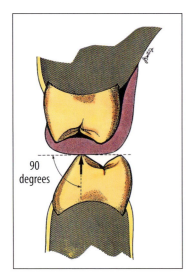

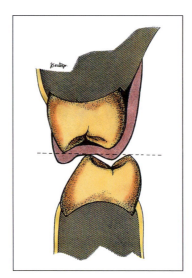

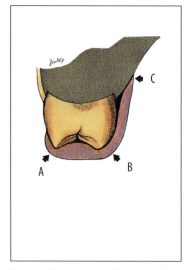

Fig 5-30 A stable relationship is achieved when the mandibular molars contact the occlusal splint, forming an angle of 90 degrees.

Fig 5-31 Amount of lateral freedom for occlusal splints with a limited amount of vertical opening. *(dotted line)* Range of possible lateral movement.

Fig 5-32 Proper finish of the external surface of the occlusal splint. (A) Correct rounding of the buccal area; (B) correct contour of the lingual area to prevent the encroachment of tongue space; (C) knife-edge finishing of the acrylic resin to provide comfort for the patient.

The vertical dimension should be inspected prior to waxing to avoid perforations; as mentioned earlier, a plane made by the tips of the mandibular molar cusps should clear the maxillary lingual cusps (Fig 5-31).

The waxup is examined and sent to the laboratory for processing. At this point, refinements of lateral and protrusive guidance can be made or altered. The waxup of the external surfaces is finished at this time. Excessive contours on the buccal area, lingual area, and borders of the wax should be avoided (Fig 5-32).

Insertion of the bite splint

The appliance should securely and comfortably adapt to the teeth and have satisfactory retention before adjustments are performed. Sometimes, a faulty impression, failure to block out undercut areas, or other problems may cause irregularities. If necessary, cold-cure acrylic resin should be removed or added. A light coating of pressure-indicating paste should be applied to the internal surface of the appliance to identify points that require adjustment. Cold-cure acrylic resin is added to the facial and lingual aspects of the appliance for extra reten-

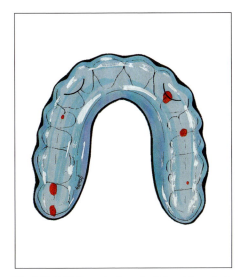

Fig 5-33 Initial examination of splint centric contacts *(red marks)* of an acrylic resin occlusal bite splint.

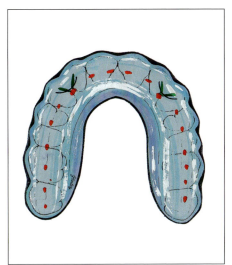

Fig 5-34 Final appearance of the occlusal contact area of the splint. All splint centric contacts have been marked *(red marks)*, and the path of anterior guidance for lateral and protrusive movements *(green lines)* is indicated.

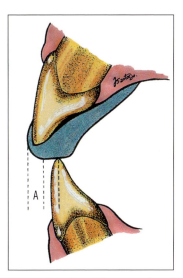

Fig 5-35 Rounding of the anterior buccal border (A) to improve speech and lip seal.

tion. Adjusting an ill-fitting appliance in the patient's mouth is time consuming and will not provide the desirable results. If the appliance does not fit well, it should be discarded and a new one should be manufactured.

The initial occlusal contacts (in splint centric) are marked with articulating ribbon, carbon paper, or 28-gauge wax (Fig 5-33). The heaviest contacts are ground the most, and all other contacts are ground to different degrees, until every opposing tooth contacts the acrylic resin with equal force (Fig 5-34).

Eccentric excursive movements are observed for interferences with the articulating ribbon or carbon paper. No marks should be produced during this maneuver. The only marks visible should be the centric stops, which should not enlarge or smudge to the sides. The only additional markings should be made by the canines during protrusive and lateral movements (see Fig 5-34).

The appearance of the appliance should be improved to enhance the patient's acceptance and cooperation. Excess acrylic resin should be removed from the anterior facial aspect of the appliance without altering its function or retention (Fig 5-35). The bulk of the buccal overlap of the appliance must not be more than 1 mm thick.

The splint is smoothed without removal of any occlusal contacts. A soft rag wheel on a lathe is used at low speed with very wet pumice to prevent heating and warping of the acrylic resin.

The patient is taught how to properly care for and use the appliance. The clinician should confirm that the patient understands the purpose of the appliance and, if necessary, give an instruction sheet to each patient at the end of the session (Box 5-1).

> **Box 5-1   Patient information about use and care of the occlusal bite splint**
>
> The occlusal bite splint you have received aids in reducing jaw muscle tension, decreasing painful symptoms, protecting the teeth, and/or maintaining the teeth in one position. Following is a list of information with helpful hints related to the use of your splint:
>
> - The splint should be worn regularly as instructed.
> - Saliva flow will increase during approximately the first 2 weeks that you wear the splint.
> - Each time the splint is placed over your teeth, it will feel somewhat tight for a few minutes.
> - Each time the splint is removed from your mouth, your "bite" may feel different for several minutes.
> - When the splint is not to be worn for more than 1 to 2 hours, it should be kept moist. Either place it in water or wrap it in a wet paper towel.
> - Regular periodic checkups are necessary to adjust and confirm the fit of your splint. If no ongoing appointments are made, do not wear your splint more than 4 to 6 months without having the fit and adjustment checked.
> - Your splint should be kept clean, just as your teeth should. Bad breath and/or bad taste may result from neglect in this area. Brush your splint with a toothbrush and toothpaste several times a day.
> - You may find it difficult to pronounce certain words when the splint is first worn. After a few days, speech will return to almost normal. Practice reading a newspaper aloud in private to help learn new speaking skills.
> - You should not continuously bite or clench on the splint. It is intended to help you relax, not exercise.

Adjustment, completion, and maintenance

After the splint is delivered, the patient should return as frequently as necessary (within a week, when possible) so that the clinician can check the splint and document the patient's progress. The clinician should investigate all problems such as tooth soreness, increase or decrease in muscle or joint tenderness, problems with speech, or any other complaint. It is especially important to note if any teeth are no longer touching the splint, for example, the anterior, posterior, right, or left dentition.

At the end of the final check of the fit of the splint, the occlusal contacts are refined in centric relation. If one or more teeth are sore where the splint is inserted, acrylic resin can be cautiously removed from the internal surface of the splint, but only in the areas where the sore teeth make excessively heavy contacts with their corresponding indentations.

Splint therapy is highly individualized. Each case will be different. The practitioner should establish the intervals for the appointments and the length of treatment with the bite splint according to the specific needs of each patient.

Use of the split-cast technique

It is possible to adjust the splint on the articulator without removing the appliance from the cast. For this process, the base of the cast must be scored with V-shaped grooves before it is mounted on the articulator. This procedure will provide a secure way to relate the cast back on the mounting plate on the articulator. Before the cast and splint are related on the articulator, all roughness and indentations are removed from the acrylic resin surface. The cast is then secured to the mounting plate with sticky wax.

After an initial check of the occlusal contacts, the occlusal surface is smoothed, preserving a flat area for opposing supporting cusps (see Fig 5-34). Each mandibular supporting cusp should contact the splint in centric occlusion (splint centric). With the condylar spheres of the articulator centered in the condylar housings, a large acrylic white stone or acrylic bur is used to adjust the surface until at least one cusp of each mandibular tooth contacts the splint. The presence of contacts is examined with articulating paper or ribbon.

Canine guidance areas should be checked and, if necessary, built up or reshaped to produce disclusion of the posterior teeth in all excursive movements. The articulator is moved in lateral excursions with the incisal pin touching the lateral wings of the incisal table. Articulating paper or ribbon is used to ensure that the opposing canine guidance produces straight lines of guidance. The splint is inspected for the presence or absence of posterior tooth contact during working- and balancing-side contacts on the surface of the acrylic resin (see Fig 5-34). During protrusive movements of the articulator, the clinician should verify that marks are being produced simultaneously in a continuous and straight line on both surfaces of each guiding ramp as well as disclusion of posterior teeth. If the guiding ramps are correct, no contacts should occur between mandibular teeth on the posterior or even anterior surfaces of the splint. Abrupt guidance should be avoided. When the articulator is moved to eccentric positions, the space created between mandibular teeth and the acrylic resin surface at the posterior segment of the dental arch must not exceed 2 mm (see Fig 5-28). The guidance is considered correct when there are V-shaped marks on the guiding ramps.

The splint is carefully removed from the cast with a knife or spatula. Any sharp areas are smoothed with an acrylic bur. The buccal surfaces are trimmed to simulate the natural tooth contours and embrasures. The splint should be no more than 1 mm thick on the buccal surfaces. The teeth should evenly touch the occlusal surface of the appliance during centric contacts and canine guidance. Patients must also have multiple contacts in centric relation as well as contacts for all mandibular supporting cusps in splint centric. This idea complies with the requirements of the freedom in centric concept when the appliance will be further adjusted in the mouth.

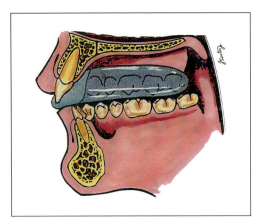

Fig 5-36 Variation of splint design. A large overjet will demand a wide anterior platform for mandibular incisors.

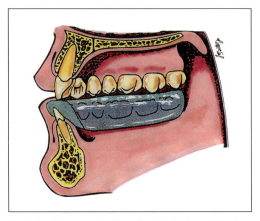

Fig 5-37 Patients with Class III malocclusion will be best served with a mandibular bite splint.

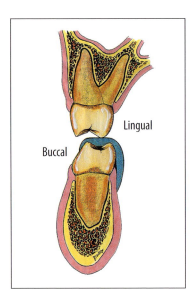

Lingual

Buccal

Fig 5-38 Molar relationship when a mandibular bite splint is fabricated.

Design modifications

The presence of excessive overjet will generate an appliance with an unusual palatal "plateau" for the incisors (Fig 5-36). Hence, the lingual extension of the appliance must be carefully contoured to prevent encroachment on the tongue space.

Cases of Class III malocclusions may represent a predicament for the fabrication of a maxillary bite splint. For patients with this condition, the best approach is to fabricate a mandibular appliance (Figs 5-37 and 5-38).

IMMEDIATE CHAIRSIDE FABRICATION

The same basic procedures are used for immediate chairside fabrication as for laboratory fabrication of bite splints, except that the appliance is directly fabricated on the cast using self-curing acrylic. The reader may therefore refer to the illustrations in the previous section for clarification.

Clinical indications

When an occlusal bite splint is urgently needed, the procedure may be carried out directly in a clinical setting. Chairside fabrication may be indicated:

- For urgent treatment of acute functional disturbances of the masticatory apparatus, trauma from occlusion, temporomandibular disorders, and so on.
- For short-term appliance therapy, such as trial diagnosis of temporomandibular disorders or prerestorative occlusal registrations.
- For protection of newly placed dental restorative work (especially porcelain reconstructions).
- As a provisional appliance, when multiple modifications are anticipated during therapy (especially concerning periodic relining and alteration of occlusal contact relationships).

Materials

The most common technique for office fabrication of an occlusal bite splint is use of autopolymerizing clear acrylic resin. Construction of splints from this type of material may present some inconveniences during fabrication, primarily due to the liberation of monomer vapors, which are toxic in a closed environment. Furthermore, in spite of the apparent time-saving procedure, the use of autopolymerizing acrylic resin involves a time-consuming process of boxing of the cast, application of powder and liquid materials, removal of the appliance from the cast, and grinding of excess polymerized acrylic resin, among other tasks.

Another material used for the fabrication of chairside immediate splints is urethane dimethacrylate, a visible light–cured polymer, which presents some advantages over self-curing acrylic and is therefore recommended for use whenever possible. In addition, new materials are being continuously presented to the dental profession. Any material available on the market today has strength and shrinkage characteristics comparable to those of heat-cured acrylic resins. Chairside fabrication of bite splints, using visible light–cured materials or any other similar material, may represent a significant contribution to treatment of occlusion and temporomandibular joint problems.[1-3]

Intraoral chairside technique

One cast is needed to fabricate the appliance. Any retentive areas of the cast (especially on the lingual side) are blocked out with either baseplate wax or fast-setting stone. All interproximal and undercut areas in the boundary of the splint must be eliminated. The outline of the external limits of the appliance is inscribed on the cast with a sharp lead pencil.

The sequence of procedures to construct a bite splint (stabilization type) starts with the preparation of a baseplate (similar to a surgical stent) directly on the patient's cast. The final step will be "perfecting" the intraoral appliance.

Prior to application of the material, the cast must be coated with some type of lubricating or releasing agent. A thin coating of the lubricant is sufficient.

A rope or plate of the material is adapted to the cast to produce a thin stent. The cast with the adapted material is placed on the turntable of a curing unit. Use of a light wand is not recommended because it will take too long to cure the material and probably will not provide a complete cure. A high-intensity light (400 to 500 nm) from a quartz halogen lamp will be able to provide the polymerization activation. To ensure proper polymerization, the material should be cured for at least 10 minutes (some modern units will take just 90 seconds to complete the cure). The baseplate material will appear yellow if it is not completely polymerized.

The polymerized baseplate is removed from the cast. All sharp edges and imperfections are removed. The borders are well trimmed and smoothed. The baseplate is now gently placed in the patient's mouth for fitting and adjustment of retention. At this stage, if necessary, some relining can be carried out using small amounts of material. After the appliance is tried in the patient's mouth, excess soft material can be removed. Light activation is started directly in the patient's mouth with a light wand. This activation must be performed for no more than 1 minute, to allow removal of the appliance from the patient's mouth while the material is still pliable. The baseplate is examined for unwanted lingual undercuts. After the removal of all sharp corners and overhangs, the appliance is again placed in the patient's mouth for final cure, using light activation for 4 minutes.

Adjustment of the anterior vertical dimension of the appliance

With the stent (baseplate) in position, separators are placed on each side of the posterior segments of the arch, to assess the thickness of the appliance. Once the vertical dimension is determined, uncured material is applied to the anterior portion of the baseplate. The patient closes his or her mouth to contact the soft material with the separators in position. The mass of material can be smoothed and then cured with a light wand.

Adjustment of the posterior vertical dimension of the appliance

Fresh material is applied to both sides of the posterior segments of the baseplate, with the anterior part providing the stop. Gross imperfections are removed. Because one of the objectives of a complete-coverage occlusal appliance is to provide an ideal occlusion, all incisal edges and supporting cusps of the opposing arch must have at least one contact in centric position and multiple bilateral posterior tooth contacts in centric relation.

Creation of anterior guidance

At this point, excursive guidance can be incorporated. In general, the opposing canines are used for anterior guidance during protrusive and lateral eccentric movements of the jaws. On each opposing guiding canine, small ramps are created at the level of the external borders of the appliance.

Final polymerization

Because it is light activated, this material can be nearly perfected prior to the polymerization. At this stage, a coat of petroleum jelly or air barrier coating must be applied to the uncured material to prevent its exposure to oxygen during the curing process.

The cast with the conforming material is placed on the turntable of a light-curing unit, or a light wand can be used. A high-intensity light from a quartz halogen lamp provides the polymerization activation. To ensure proper polymerization, the cast must be left in the curing unit for at least 10 minutes. The bite splint will appear yellow if it is not completely polymerized.

Extraoral chairside technique

The following technique employs the use of two casts mounted in the articulator. This method is convenient for the fabrication of any model of bite splint; personal experience of the clinician should dictate the choice of using one or two casts. Although any type of simple hinge articulator can be used, it is advisable to mount the casts on a semiadjustable articulator. This procedure may reduce the amount of time necessary to adjust the occlusal splint at chairside. Following the completion of mounting procedures, the bite splint fabrication can be carried out directly on the articulator. The appliance may be fabricated for the maxilla or mandible, according to clinical indications. The procedures for fabrication will be similar to those described for intraoral fabrication. For the sake of simplification, an example of maxillary occlusal bite splint construction (stabilization type) will be described, although many types of designs can be made.

Mounting of casts on the articulator

The mounting of the casts on the articulator must always follow the manufacturer's instructions. A centric relation wax record may be used to mount the mandibular cast on the articulator. However, in some clinical circumstances, the proper manipulation of the mandible in centric relation is not always possible. If the patient has symptoms that impede correct manipulation, casts may be mounted in maximum intercuspation (centric occlusion). Protrusive or lateral checkbite recordings are then utilized to set the condylar guidance.

Fabrication

The fabrication of the appliance begins with the selection of the appropriate dental arch. In some clinical cases, depending on the number of teeth available and the position and extension of edentulous spaces, the tendency is to select the arch that will be able to provide the best retention and stability for the future appliance. After the arch has been selected, the outline of the splint is drawn on the cast and retentive areas are blocked out (especially on the lingual side) with either baseplate wax or fast-setting stone.

The vertical dimension is adjusted on the articulator so that the intercuspal distance between the last molars of the opposing casts is increased to at least 2 mm.

The cast is coated with lubricating media. A thin coating of the lubricating agent is sufficient. The opposing cast is also coated on the occlusal thirds of the teeth.

A rope or sheet of plastic material is used to form the body of the splint. The sheet is adapted and trimmed to the previously outlined cast. Sometimes just one layer of material is enough to fabricate the appliance. The unused scraps of material should always be saved. Material is added, as needed, to the occlusal surface and to construct the anterior guidance. The unused material must always be protected against exposure to any source of light to prevent the initiation of polymerization.

The casts are then articulated on the closed articulator. The occlusal relationships of the splint are developed. Surgical gloves should always be worn by the operator during these procedures; all indentations can be smoothed with the fingers (lubricated with separating media). Before additional layers of the material are applied, a thin coat of bonding substance must be applied to the raw surface of the appliance.

Usually, opposing canines are used for anterior guidance in protrusive and in lateral eccentric movements of the jaws. At the level of each opposing guiding canine, small ramps are created on the external borders of the appliance. Steep guidance should be avoided. All edges of the ramps are then rounded. Before polymerization is started, the casts are articulated and the guiding ramps are checked for accuracy.

The material on the cast is allowed to cure in a unit for 10 minutes. If the material still displays a yellowish appearance, an extra 5 to 10 minutes of polymerization should be added to complete the cure. A protective substance (petroleum jelly or an air barrier coating) must be used to prevent contact of the material with air during the curing process. When polymerization is completed, the cast is removed from the turntable and the splint is gently removed from the cast. If wax was used as a block-out material, the softened wax is peeled out of the splint while the wax is still warm.

The splint is returned to the cast, the cast is placed back on the articulator, and all centric contacts are adjusted. All eccentric interferences are eliminated. Articulating ribbon is used to examine all contacts in splint centric and to check if all of them are uniform. Splint centric is a position achieved when the patient bites on the appliance. If not, the splint must be readjusted. The continuity of the canine guidance must be examined.

The fit and retention of the splint are confirmed. Internal adjustment and relining may be needed if the appliance is not stable in the mouth.

After the initial fabrication phase, articulating ribbon with different colors is used once more to check for occlusal contacts in the patient's mouth. Any interference is eliminated, and the anterior guidance is improved. Eventually, more adjustments may be performed before the appliance is delivered.

The splint is finished and polished to a high shine using pumice. The final result will be a translucent, hard bite splint that needs minimal intraoral adjustment when inserted in the patient's mouth.

If additive corrections are needed, the surface of the bite splint is roughened with an acrylic stone and coated with a bonding agent. Then sufficient visible light–cured material is added to complete the necessary occlusal corrections. The additional splint material must be adequately cured.

Advantages of chairside fabrication

- The most important advantage is the ability to visualize the final splint prior to polymerization.
- The appliance may be fabricated and delivered in the same appointment. This is especially important in cases of acute trauma, when the patient is suffering pain and dysfunction.
- This method provides the ability to produce different designs, including anterior plateaus, deprogramming devices, and complete-coverage appliances (with or without anterior guidance).
- There is limited involvement of laboratory work in the production of the appliances.
- This technique reduces the time and expense of fabrication.
- Proper corrections, repairs, finishing, and polishing are easily accomplished.
- There is no exposure to free monomer.

Disadvantages of chairside fabrication

- Care must be exerted to provide a completely cured material before the appliance is delivered. Uncured material may have a bad taste. The patient should be instructed to keep the appliance in mouthwash during the first week to prevent a bad taste.
- Relining may be troublesome, because contact with soft tissues in the mouth must be avoided.
- The long-term translucency of the cured material is unknown at present.
- Very thin appliances (less than 1 mm thick) have a tendency to be brittle. Fabrication of bite splints with limited thickness is contraindicated.

REFERENCES

1. dos Santos J Jr, Park JG, Re GJ. Patient preference between visible light-cured and heat-cured acrylic splints. Am J Dent 2000;13:305–307.
2. dos Santos J Jr, Gurklis M. Chairside fabrication of occlusal biteplane splints using visible light cured materials. Cranio 1995;13:131–126.
3. dos Santos J Jr, Gurklis M. Immediate fabrication of occlusal bitesplints using visible light-cured material. Compendium 1994;15:228–232.

CONSERVATIVE TREATMENT OF TEMPOROMANDIBULAR DISORDERS

This chapter will suggest modalities of conservative treatment, which may be used as support for other forms of conventional therapy for temporomandibular disorders (TMDs). In general, the dental professional can count on physical and pharmacologic agents[1-5] for pain control among these modalities of treatment. Physical agents include applications of heat and cold,[6] massage, mobilization, immobilization, and therapeutic exercises.[7] Examples of pharmacologic agents are analgesics, anti-inflammatories, muscle relaxants,[8] tranquilizers, anticonvulsives, vasoactives, anesthetic injections, and unguents.

Acute conditions demand urgent management; however, the use of these modalities is also indicated for chronic cases. Compresses, exercises, and some medications are commonly employed in dentistry and are clearly indicated for symptomatic relief of long-lasting orofacial pain.

PHYSICAL AGENTS

Physical agents used for the treatment of TMDs include a great variety of procedures and indications. Some modalities may be used as an adjunct to other treatment for symptomatic control.

Cold and heat

Cold and heat[6] are used to placate pain, acting directly on the peripheral innervation of the masticatory system, especially at the level of free nerve endings, producing a counterirritant effect. Studies pertaining to the effects of temperature on muscle spindles have demonstrated that afferent neurotransmission of group IA fibers increases with heat and decreases with cold.[6] The physiologic foundation for the relief of muscle spasm with the use of temperature is not yet clear. Muscle spasm is usually the secondary result of neuropathology or skeletal muscle dysfunction.

Another physiologic response is an increased blood flow with the use of heat and a tendency for ischemia with the use of cold. The combination of heat (as vasodilator agent) and cold may be helpful in the treatment of a great number of clinical cases.

Cryotherapy (cold therapy)

Cold has the property of reducing muscle excitability and spasm. The beneficial result of the use of cold in cases of muscle spasm is reduction of muscle spindle response to stretch reflex reactions.

In contact sports or car accidents, pain from direct trauma may be alleviated, and to a certain degree even prevented, by the immediate application of cold compresses. Because of its vasoconstrictive effect, cold not only reduces pain perception but also prevents formation of edema.

The masticatory system of a patient who has been exposed to nonfunctional activity, such as unaccustomed chewing, excessive mouth opening during yawning, or extrinsic or intrinsic injury to joints and muscles, suffers strained connective tissue. In this case, all evidence indicates that the collagen, the most abundant protein in the human body and the most important constituent of the fibrous connective tissue, suffers elastic deformation beyond its tolerance capacity.[6] The prescription of a treatment capable of recovering this elastic property is indicated. The application of cold is definitely indicated in these cases. It has the ability to increase the stiffness of collagen and consequently reduce the deformity of the fibers (tendons and ligaments).

There are numerous modalities of treatment using cryotherapy. Among those used in dentistry are ice bags, cold packs, and cooling sprays of ethyl chloride or chlorofluormethane (nonflammable). Commercially available cold packs or plastic bags with ice can be used as cold compresses. They are applied directly on the afflicted site.

In cases of spasm and limitation of movements, superficial application of cooling sprays is used to interrupt the vicious circle of pain. They have been considered a fast and efficient way of providing symptomatic treatment, but their effect is of short duration. During application of the spray, it is beneficial to produce movements of the parts being treated. This treatment is not as effective for chronic pain.

In addition to its analgesic effect, cold reduces local blood circulation. Inflammatory responses, edema, or even hemorrhage are diminished. Low temperature, as used superficially, has been demonstrated to be helpful in reducing pain and increasing mandibular mobility,[6] but it is advisable to use it in combination with active exercise therapy.

If reduction of muscle spasm is one of the objectives of treatment, the use of cold during a session of application must continue for at least 20 minutes. Acute inflammatory response following a traumatic injury such as intense muscle or joint distension should be treated by application of cold for 15 or 20 minutes with 30-minute intervals several times a day. In subacute or chronic injury, applications are carried out for 30 minutes twice a day. Although cold is indicated for treating traumatic lesions, it is not advisable to use it for more than 48 hours, because it may interfere with the healing process.[6]

Patients with degenerative temporomandibular joint conditions must not be exposed to local cold applications because the stiffness produced by low temperatures may increase the symptoms.

Unfavorable effects resulting from applications of low temperature are unusual and generally related to hypersensitivity to cold. An example of hypersensitivity to superficial cooling may be the development of a rash, because of local release of histamine-like substances from tissues underlying the skin.

Thermotherapy (heat therapy)

The elevation of temperature at the site of pathosis may generate different responses:

- Changes in neuromuscular activity related to its depressing effect on muscle fibers.
- Capillary arteriolar dilation causing an increase in blood flow. This effect is the result of a great concentration of carbon dioxide, which causes vessel dilation.
- Increase of local enzymatic activity. The increase of blood carries away catabolite, bringing greater supply of nutrients and blood-healing elements (antibodies, leukocytes, etc) to provide phagocytosis.
- Alterations in pain threshold mainly because of the sedative effect of heat application, a mechanism not yet well understood.

Clinical cases involving masticatory muscle tension, pain, and stiffness of temporomandibular joints (especially in patients with rheumatoid arthritis or ankylosis) may benefit because of vigorous reactions to heat therapy.

The elasticity of collagen tissue is increased in the presence of heat. The viscous flow of fibers increases, resulting in relaxation of their tensional properties and producing a residual elongation. The physiologic mechanism that produces reduction of pain with temperature elevation is probably at the level of the cellular function of vital tissues.

It is possible that the increase of local temperature at the spastic muscle may reduce its sensitivity to stretch, thus relieving the spasm.

The increased vascularity resulting from heat is important in relieving pain in myositis and fibrositis. These pathologic states, which do not represent defined syndromes, have favorable responses to the increase in temperature at painful trigger points emerging in superficial areas of the body. The response to the application of heat to treat inflammation is also beneficial.

Superficial heat
Hot, moist compresses and dry, radiant heat are the most commonly used agents for this type of therapy.

Hot, moist compresses
To produce the desired result, hot, moist compresses must be used for no less than 20 minutes three or more times a day. The patient should avoid being exposed to outside cold temperature after each application. Hot, moist compresses may be used by patients at home. The heat is obtained by immersing a towel in hot water at a bearable temperature, removing excess moisture and applying to both sides of the face (Fig 6-1), avoiding scalding of the skin. A wet towel can also be heated in a home microwave oven. It has been established that the use of an automatic moist heating pad provides additional gain compared to conventional hot, moist applications.[9] It is possible that the control of heat and its ease of application may offer added advantages in terms of patient compliance with the prescribed treatment.

Hot, moist compresses have been generally preferred over dry, radiant heat because there is less risk of burning the skin.

Heat therapy should not be chosen for the following conditions or individuals:

- Areas of localized hemorrhage
- Acute cases of thrombophlebitis
- Areas of malignant tumors
- Infants or elderly individuals
- Patients with partial facial anesthesia
- Cases of extensive trauma

Deep heat
The therapeutic use of deep heat produces increased temperature localized distant from the affected site, and the response is less intense. Deep heat is generated by special instruments:

- Microwaves: electromagnetic radiation in the range of 915 to 2,456 MHz
- Shortwave diathermy: high-frequency electromagnetic currents operating at the level of 27.12 MHz
- Ultrasound: high-frequency acoustic vibrations in the range of 0.8 to 1.0 MHz
- Soft (low-level) laser: radiation emitted by gallium-aluminum-arsenic with 830-nm wavelength

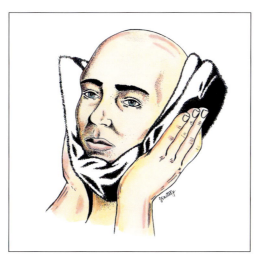

Fig 6-1 A wet towel is used as a moist heat compress. The towel is applied to both sides of the face for better results.

Because of the localized increase of temperature, microwave diathermy should not be used in the proximity of metallic dental restorations. Disregarding this precaution may be highly damaging to the patient.

None of these agents producing nonthermal heat have been proved to be essential for symptomatic therapy, in spite of having a great deal of heat infiltration. Moreover, some of them may even present some risks to the patient, although some of the effects are not considered destructive.[9] Application of microwaves, for example, may produce a "pearl necklace" of corpuscles inside of the bloodstream; however, danger from this effect has not been documented. This kind of pearl necklace may also be produced with shortwave diathermy. These instruments must not be used in areas adjacent to the brain and eyes. Ultrasound, for instance, may produce interstitial tissue gaseous cavitations, mainly inside temporomandibular joints and ocular orbs.[9]

There are two modalities of laser: hard and soft. For treatment of TMDs, the soft or low-level laser constitutes a modality of treatment where the therapeutic effect is mainly the result of light absorption rather than the result of local increase of skin temperature. Therefore, this type of laser can generate internal tissue changes, leading to favorable metabolic cell activations. In this way, it creates an anti-inflammatory reaction within the damaged tissues of joints and muscles, leading to a healing process and elimination of pain. It is believed that this process may be useful for treatment of, among others, chronic pains; rheumatoid arthritis; neuralgias; myofascial pain; and fibromyalgia. However, no long-term scientific studies have demonstrated the effective action of this treatment modality.

Therapeutic exercises

Therapeutic exercises use the contraction of masticatory muscles that promote mandibular movement in such a way that the patient becomes the main agent during the treatment. Some clinicians consider therapeutic exercises to be necessary for the resolution of residual subclinical stages of TMD and even for the prevention of future cases of dysfunction. Therapeutic exercises are considered relevant for the functional recuperation of the masticatory system, even when complications involving cervical structures are considered. Because of the great diversity of exercises available, it is possible to choose the most suitable to be used in dentistry, including assisted muscular stretching, stretching against resistance, and resistance against opening or closing.

Assisted muscular stretching

This type of exercise consists of isotonic contractions intended for patient reeducation in the use of the masticatory musculature. It is always accomplished by smooth and symmetric opening and closing motions of the mandible, without producing any discomfort.

These maneuvers are carried out by the patient, who is advised to use both the forefinger and thumb of one hand resting against the incisal edge of maxillary and mandibular incisors. Using digital force, the patient tries to open the mouth (Fig 6-2). The movement produced approaches the hinge axis of the mandible. More extensive translational movements may be tried later. The sequence of operations is carried out three to four times daily. This exercise is instituted to activate the pterygoid muscles, especially the bilateral external pterygoid muscles (Fig 6-3).

Stretching against resistance

The isotonic action produced by this exercise represents an extension of the previously described maneuver. The contraction of mandibular depressor muscles against resistance, in this series of exercises, facilitates the inhibitory action on the mandibular elevator muscles, especially in cases of muscle splinting. The patient's fist provides resistance during symmetric mandibular opening (Fig 6-4). This exercise is also known as *reflex relaxation* of the mandibular elevator muscles (Fig 6-5). This exercise is repeated three to four times daily.

This exercise should not be used in patients with chronic morphologic and degenerative alteration of the temporomandibular joints. There are other modalities of treatment that maintain movement of the mandible during functional therapy without delivering substantial stress to the internal structures of the joints. Exercises

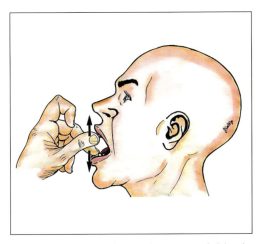

Fig 6-2 Assisted muscular stretching is provided by the patient's fingers. In this case, the thumb and forefinger rest on the mandibular and maxillary incisors to provide controlled opening of the jaw *(arrows)*.

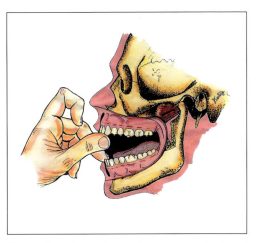

Fig 6-3 Assisted muscular stretching produces activation of the pterygoid group of muscles.

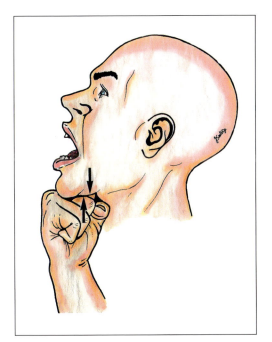

Fig 6-4 The masticatory muscles are stretched against resistance provided by the patient's fist. In this case, an opening action of the jaw is opposed by the patient's fist *(arrows)*.

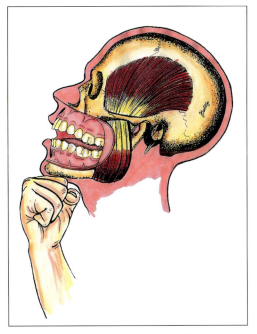

Fig 6-5 Stretching against resistance provides activation of elevator muscles (masseter and temporalis).

should be avoided in patients with internal adhesions in the joints and ankylosis. The use of occlusal bite splints and, when indicated, surgical intervention should be considered as alternatives.

Resistance against closing or opening

This type of exercise is accomplished by mobilizing the elevator and depressor musculature of the jaws against resistance. This type of procedure is useful when attempting to break the vicious circle of muscular splinting or spasm.

This series of maneuvers may be performed by the patient or by the therapist (Fig 6-6). The routine consists of trying to move the mandible against the bracing action of the patient's fist or the professional's hands. In this circumstance, the masticatory muscles will produce strong isometric contraction without any movement of the parts. Each set of exercises is repeated four times daily.

When the acute condition subsides completely, the patient is then directed to move the jaw in other functional pathways. It is necessary to prescribe a soft diet and tell the patient to avoid extended chewing during this period of treatment; likewise, extensive movements should be avoided.

To avoid undesirable results, the professional must instruct the patient in the use of exercises. Beginning with slow, short, smooth movements, the patient may gradually increase the intensity of the maneuvers to produce a wider range of motion. Some rules must be observed:

* Perform with regularity: The series should be continued on a regular basis.
* Limit repetitions: The patient should avoid performing excessive repetitions in a short period of time, which may produce painful motions, leading to stiffness of muscle and joints.
* Avoid fatigue: The patient should not extend the number of exercises to the point where pain will be elicited.

Continuous passive motion

There are some claims that continuous passive motion is becoming a widely accepted modality of treatment for orthopedic rehabilitation of the temporomandibular joint, especially after surgery of the joint.[7,10]

During the procedure for passive motion, minute, continuous, and controlled translational movement is imparted to the articular surfaces, through the action of occlusal plates, which produces horizontal motion. During the application of the device, the patient is able to control the increase of speed and range of motion.

Because adhesion of the joints may be the result of any type of invasive joint surgery, the objectives for the use of these devices are inhibition of contracture by synthesis of glycosaminoglycans, which is able to maintain lubrication and redirect

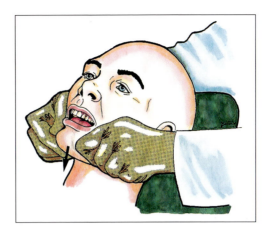

Fig 6-6 Resistance against opening or closing of the jaw *(arrow)* provided by the therapist.

formation of collagen fibers; improvement of fluid dynamics inside the joint under surgery; stimulation of mechanoreceptors to relieve pain through a modulating effect of thick fibers; prevention of the formation of adhesions; and prevention of muscle atrophy (if the joints are kept immobilized for a long period of time).

Electrical stimulation

This modality of treatment has been proposed in dentistry in recent years. The most frequently suggested technique is transcutaneous electric nerve stimulation.[9–11] In dentistry, it is utilized at the level of the peripheral nociceptive receptors. This practice, praised by clinicians, is a productive way to control neurogenic and masticatory muscle pains, because the temporary activation of afferent nerves by transcutaneous neural stimulation modulates pain. Stimulation of peripheral nerves (or even other structures along the brain stem) is able to produce pain relief. This mechanism is not totally understood; however, there are some latent areas along the neural pathway between the stimulating site and the brain stem where pain modulation could originate.

There is no definite confirmation that the central nervous system is directly involved in the mechanism of pain control in this case. Certainly, the primary site to be stimulated would be the peripheral receptors. At this site, there may be a blocking effect of the action potential of A-delta fibers.[10,11]

Another theory considers that local stimulation excites distant neurons along the central pathways in the brain, propagating a peripheral inhibitory action. In this case, the inhibitory effect is accounted for by neurophysiologic activity or is due to the liberation of neurotransmitter substances (for example, serotonin).[9–11]

Instrumentation

Superficial electrodes are used to convey electronic impulses through the skin to the area under treatment (Fig 6-7). In general, one dispersing and two active electrodes are used. They are fabricated from special high-conductance metallic alloys (silver–silver chloride, for example) and are part of the instrumentation hardware for stimulation.

Placement of the active electrodes conform to the neurologic sites of the orofacial regions to be activated. The electrodes are positioned to incorporate muscle motor endplates, which constitute areas corresponding to sensitive and motor free nerve endings, and/or muscle trigger points.

Amount and duration

The amount and duration of stimulation must be well supervised by the therapist. The dental professional counts on technical or auxiliary personnel to help in the use of the instrumentation for electrostimulation; therefore, special training is required. Initial applications are carried out above the neurologic threshold level, for an average of 1-hour duration for each session and, in critical cases, three to four times a day. When patients are familiarized with the use of the instrument, they can adjust the best level of stimulation for their own use.

In the beginning, the amount of stimulation may be adjusted as follows:

- Pulse: 2-millisecond duration and 1.5-second interval
- Frequency: between 0 and 100 Hz
- Voltage: current of 60 mA, from 0 to 90 V
- Use: 15 minutes to 1 hour

To avoid an indefinite application of the stimulation, it is necessary to follow some parameters:

- Effective time: The effective time for the initiation of analgesia is defined to be the amount of time that has elapsed from the beginning of each session to the instant the patient reveals eradication of pain.
- Effect duration: This parameter is defined by the interval between the instant the stimulus is discontinued until the recurrence of pain.
- Effective gain: This demarcation is measured by the difference between the effective time for the installation of the analgesia and the duration of the stimulation effect. The greater the difference, the better will be the results of the therapy.

Fig 6-7 Electrical stimulation. Electrode placement to provide stimulation to selected areas is shown. (F) Frontalis muscle and supraorbital branch of the ophthalmic division of the trigeminal nerve; (T) upper zygomatic branches of the trigeminal, facial nerves, and temporalis muscle; (J) temporomandibular joint, sigmoid notch, and auriculotemporal nerve; (M) masseter muscle and sensory branches of facial and trigeminal nerves.

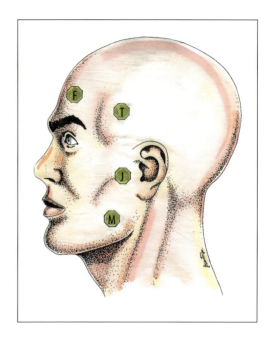

Low-frequency stimulation

During this type of stimulation, low-frequency (2-Hz) impulses with currents of high intensity (up to the level of 90 V and 60 mA) are generated with a frequency of 1 to 2 impulses per second and may produce analgesic action. The excitation is more effective when applied to muscle nociceptives (afferent fibers of groups III and IV) that, in turn, activate the antinociceptive endogenous system.

The onset of the action is felt after an induction phase of 15 to 20 minutes' duration. The analgesia may reach segmental divisions or the entire body. Segmental pain reduction occurs due to enkephalin liberation, while whole-body pain modulation is caused by the hormonal action of endorphins (originated at the level of the pituitary glands and carried by the blood flow).

This kind of stimulation involves specific points considered "acupuncture points." Therefore, analgesia with the use of low-frequency stimulation is also used in electroacupuncture. One of the most recent achievements in this field is related to the use of a cold laser (helium-neon) directly applied to acupuncture points of the body. This procedure, although its use is incipient in the dental profession, seems to provide more effective and less sensitive acupuncture stimulations than conventional acupuncture.[9–11]

High-frequency stimulation

During high-frequency stimulation, each pulse has the duration of 2 milliseconds with 0.5- to 1.5- second intervals. The voltage is low, barely exceeding 4 V.

The effect of this kind of stimulation is instantaneous and confined to the excited location; there are no reports of side effects. It is apparent that the analgesic effect is quite efficient, reducing the pain from 50% to 70%, but the effect is of short duration.[9–11]

Local burning, slight prickling, or needling sensations can be experienced when the intensity of the current used for stimulation is increased. Advancements in the production of new instruments now tend to prevent this annoyance. In addition, this stimulation may start to produce rhythmic contraction of adjacent muscles in synchrony with the continuous excitation.

The use of high-frequency transcutaneous neural stimulation (square waves in the range of 50- to 100-Hz impulses), but at low intensity, is very efficient in inhibiting pain.[9–11] This variety of current stimulates A-beta cutaneous afferent fibers, which in turn may mobilize the inhibitory descending mechanism, without receiving any direct influence of the opiate peptide of the nervous system (enkephalins and/or endorphins).

PHARMACOLOGIC AGENTS

Most pharmacologic agents are used to control chronic pain afflicting the orofacial regions; however, this does not mean that there are no indications for their uses in acute cases. To define indications and contraindications, incompatibilities to drugs, side effects, complications, and so on, it is important to clearly identify the clinical problem.

Analgesics

In general, analgesics are divided into three main groups: anti-inflammatory nonnarcotics (Table 6-1), nonsteroidal anti-inflammatory drugs (Table 6-2), and narcotics (Table 6-3).

The purpose in the use of analgesics is to alleviate painful conditions; however, the clinician should not expect total eradication of the patient's pain. Some professionals believe that the least amount of drug prescription should be used to prevent the exacerbation of pain.

Table 6-1 Prescription information for nonnarcotic analgesics

Medication	Maximum adult daily dosage	Indications and uses	Contraindications	Side effects
Aspirin*	4000 mg	Analgesic, anti-inflammatory, antipyretic	Ulcer, liver conditions, gouty arthritis, diabetes, asthma	Gastric problems, prolonged bleeding
Acetaminophen	4000 mg	Analgesic, allergy to aspirin	Cases of intense pain	Hepatotoxicity in overdose

*Also a nonsteroidal anti-inflammatory drug.

Table 6-2 Prescription information for nonsteroidal anti-inflammatory drugs

Medication	Maximum adult daily dosage	Indications and uses	Contraindications	Side effects
Ibuprofen	3200 mg	Analgesic, anti-inflammatory, rheumatoid arthritis, degenerative joint disease	Bleeding disorders	Gastrointestinal disturbances; may produce central nervous system effects (headaches, dizziness, vertigo, visual and auditory disturbances, etc)
Fenoprofen	3200 mg			
Naproxen	1250 mg			
Sulindac	400 mg			
Tolmetin	1800 mg			
Indomethacin	200 mg	Potent anti-inflammatory, antipyretic, analgesic, rheumatoid arthritis, ankylosis, bursitis, tendonitis	Tendency to serious toxicity	Gastrointestinal disturbances and lesions; central nervous system effects (headaches and confusion)

Table 6-3 Prescription information for narcotic analgesics

Medication	Maximum adult daily dosage	Indications and uses	Contraindications	Side effects
Codeine	360 mg	Analgesic (oral), antitussive	None	Dependence; non–anti-inflammatory action; central nervous system effects (nausea, dizziness, sedation)
Propoxylene	390 mg	Analgesic	None	Dependence; central nervous system effects (depression, convulsion, hallucination)
Oxycodone	30 mg	Analgesic	None	May produce dependence
Meperedine	300 mg	Potent analgesic, sedative	Respiratory depression	Central nervous system effects (tremor, convulsion, dependence)

Anti-inflammatory nonnarcotic analgesics

Anti-inflammatory nonnarcotic drugs consist of a heterogenous group of chemicals that are effective in the treatment of pain arising from an inflammatory process. The sequence of reactions leading to the synthesis of prostaglandin is entirely associated with the local inflammatory response, producing the sensitivity of peripheral nerve endings. The efficiency of these medications in the treatment of painful states caused by inflammatory processes is closely associated with the inhibition of prostaglandin synthesis.

The most common complication of the constant use of these substances is to gastric ulcerations, although current products on the market claim the correction of this problem. Patients with hypersensitivity to these substances may present with significant life-threatening allergies.

Conventional over-the-counter pharmacologic preparations are represented by various brands of aspirin and acetaminophen.

Aspirin
Aspirin is the most frequently prescribed substance in this class of agents. In cases of severe inflammatory processes, this drug is used in high dosages. However, in less critical conditions, aspirin in smaller dosages can be prescribed with relative success. Aspirin belongs to the widespread chemical class of salicylate and is synthesized as acetylsalicylic acid.

The anti-inflammatory property of aspirin may be of some benefit for rapid pain control because of its analgesic effect, but it is incorrect to assume that the analgesic effect is exclusively due to the anti-inflammatory property of this drug. This drug is used for almost all painful conditions.

Aspirin may initiate some blood changes by extending the bleeding time, owing to the inhibition of platelet aggregation.

Acetaminophen
Acetaminophen is customarily prescribed as a replacement for aspirin. Although its anti-inflammatory property is not as significant, its action is similar to aspirin. Acetaminophen has fewer side effects than aspirin, but when used in high dosages acetaminophen can cause irreversible liver complications (hepatotoxicity). This type of analgesic does not inhibit platelet aggregation, unlike aspirin. This drug became commercially successful in the mid-1900s and was synthesized from aniline derivatives with antipyretic properties.

Nonsteroidal anti-inflammatory drugs

Although aspirin is also included in this category and seems to be the precursor of all medications included in this category, there are some other substances used in dentistry that present added characteristics of anti-inflammatory/nonnarcotic substances. The most frequently used are ibuprofen and naproxen sodium. Those less frequently used are indomethacin; fenoprofen; sulindac; and tolmetin. In general these drugs have many more side effects than aspirin or acetaminophen.

Narcotic analgesics

These analgesics are morphine-like substances capable of releasing endogenous opiate peptide in different levels of the nervous system.[12,13] The use of narcotics in dentistry is almost always unsatisfactory because of the utilization and selection of inappropriate drugs. A common mistake is to prescribe a drug of rapid action and short duration for a long period of time. In this case, the patient will require a continuous increase of its use to produce the same response.

In dentistry, there are few valid reasons to prescribe such substances. Some dental professionals in hospital settings may be involved with terminally ill patients, who for legitimate reasons need immediate relief of pain.

The prescription of drugs of this nature will require careful and constant medical supervision because these substances are too easily abused. The prescription of morphine, for example, may lead to a serious addiction to the drug, which in the majority of cases may take only 10 days to develop.

In dentistry, opiate preparations such as codeine (the one most commonly used), propoxyphene, oxycodone, and meperidine may be prescribed in combination with some anti-inflammatory nonnarcotic analgesics to potentiate their actions. Pain relief is more efficient because both central and peripheral mechanisms of analgesia are involved.

Anti-inflammatories

Steroidal agents

Anti-inflammatory properties are related to biosynthesis of prostaglandin inhibition. Anti-inflammatory substances may produce increased and variable metabolic reactions, including induction of changes in the organic immunologic responses of the body. For these reasons, although useful in some cases, these drugs must be administered with care and good judgment. Although some nonsteroidal analgesic drugs can be used to control inflammatory processes, as described earlier, certain adrenal corticosteroids and their synthetic analogs are broadly used in medicine because of their efficacious anti-inflammatory action.

When acting in the suppression of inflammatory processes, corticosteroids may increase susceptibility to infections. Therefore, prolonged used of these drugs is contraindicated, especially in the presence of herpetic, bacterial, and fungal infections.

Table 6-4	Prescription information for muscle relaxants			
Medication	Maximum adult daily dosage	Indications and uses	Contraindications	Side effects
Methocarbamol	6 g	Centrally induced muscle relaxation, long-acting	None	Central nervous system effects (drowsiness, dizziness, ataxia, nystagmus, etc)
Diazepam	40 mg	Centrally induced muscle relaxation, reduction of postoperative trismus	None	Dependence; central nervous system effects (mood depression, paradoxical excitement, lethargy, etc)

In dentistry, these products may be used to control pulpal hypersensitivity, to lessen postoperative complications from edema and trismus, to treat a variety of ulcerative lesions of the oral cavity, and to reduce inflammation in temporomandibular joints. The most commonly employed agents for these purposes are hydrocortisone and prednisolone.

Nonsteroidal antihyperuricemic agents

Besides corticosteroids, there are some nonsteroidal antihyperuricemic agents that are used to control systemic temporomandibular joint problems caused by hyperuricemia (ie, gout). However, the prescription of agents such as colchinine, probenicid, allupurinol, and others is more properly the jurisdiction of medical specialists.

Muscle relaxants

Muscle-relaxing drugs act directly at the level of skeletal muscles because of selective action of the chemical at the level of the central nervous system (Table 6-4). Centrally induced muscle relaxation is primarily due to the partial suppression of tonic flow of nerve impulses to voluntary (striated) muscles. When the medications are used appropriately, the patient does not lose consciousness.

The most significant preparations in this group of muscle relaxants include methocarbamol, chlorphenesin carbamate, and clorzoxazone. All of these drugs relax skeletal muscles through a depressing effect on the central nervous system.

Another drug is orphenadrine citrate, an antihistamine analog. Its action is different from the aforementioned group, because it tends to relax the skeletal musculature and to have some value in cases of painful dysfunction of masticatory muscles. This drug has an anticholinergic effect, producing different physical symptoms such as drowsiness and sedation, and must be prescribed under medical supervision.

Benzodiazepines represent another group of muscle relaxants, of which the principal representative is diazepam. This group of compounds has a more sedative property than some centrally inducing muscle relaxants. There are some reports indicating that they provide equivalent or better muscle-relaxing outcomes with lower toxicity.[8] Diazepam seems to be the medication of choice in dentistry because it has been found to reduce postoperative trismus and may be prescribed as complement to other treatment for temporomandibular disorders.

Numerous other compounds for muscle relaxation are available. Because the centrally induced effect of muscle-relaxing drugs on peripheral muscle tone is not totally known, prudence is necessary when these medications are prescribed.

Anesthetic blocking

Anesthetic blocking is based on the interruption of the vicious circle of pain, allowing for temporary absence of pain to provide conditions for the recovery of the masticatory system. In general, injections are applied at the level of the masticatory musculature (intramuscularly and extramuscularly) and in the temporomandibular joints. The injection of anesthetics, steroids, sclerosing solutions, and hyaluronidase solutions into affected zones is a treatment approach that may notably alleviate painful conditions. However, there are some limitations in their uses, because special training is required from the therapist.

Intramuscular injections

The most commonly selected anesthetic solutions for this technique are lidocaine 1% without epinephrine or procaine 0.5% without epinephrine. It is critical to use anesthetic solutions without a vasoconstrictor to prevent prolonged action of the anesthetic or even unexpected degeneration of the muscle from localized ischemia.

To obtain the best results, some clinicians recommend infiltration of the solution directly into painful nodes (trigger zones) of the muscle. The application of superficial coolant sprays on the area to be injected is advisable, because increased discomfort for the patient is anticipated.

For the intramuscular technique, masticatory muscles are injected through the skin extraorally; however, some muscles such as the lateral pterygoid may be injected intraorally if the patient can open the mouth enough (Fig 6-8). In this case, the needle is introduced behind the maxillary tuberosity into the gingival groove (Fig 6-9). In patients with restricted opening of the mouth, the only alternative is to inject extraorally through the sigmoid notch of the mandible (Fig 6-10).

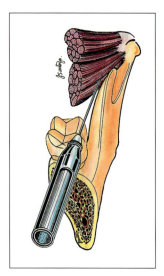

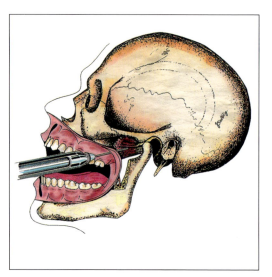

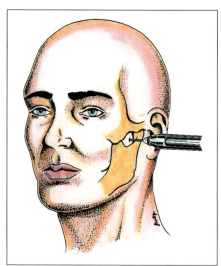

Fig 6-8 The needle direction for intraoral intramuscular injection of the anesthetic solution at the level of the pterygoid window is shown.

Fig 6-9 The intramuscular injection reaches the pterygoid window through the oral mucosa behind the molar tuberosity.

Fig 6-10 The extraoral intramuscular injection of anesthetic solution through the mandibular sigmoid notch aims at the pterygoid window. This approach is used when the patient has limited opening of the mouth.

Extramuscular injections

The selection of anesthetic solutions is the same as for the intramuscular technique. This procedure is predominately indicated in cases of masticatory elevator muscle spasms (trismus) where there is some restriction of mouth opening. This technique is less distressing and less annoying to the patient than intramuscular injections.

Commonly, it is done intraorally with the purpose of reaching the masseter or pterygoid muscles. For the masseter muscles, the needle penetrates perpendicular to the mandibular ascending ramus, approaching the muscle from its anterior border and running perpendicular to its external fibers (Figs 6-11 and 6-12). Anesthesia of the muscle results in a short period of time. When the masseter is anesthetized, a great part of the symptoms is alleviated, and the injection even diminishes the symptoms of neighboring muscles.

Although the needle for anesthetic solution injection is external to the mass of the muscle, it is important to remember that the procedure is not simple and demands good training. The presence of other anatomic structures adjacent to the area being injected must be carefully observed and evaluated (eg, parotid gland, buccinator muscle, nerves, and blood vessels).

Extramuscular injection of the external pterygoid muscle also may be performed. A long injection needle penetrates the maxillary tuberosity and reaches

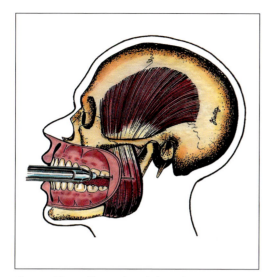

Fig 6-11 The needle goes through the oral mucosa and reaches the external outer surface of the muscle perpendicular to the mass of the masseter muscle for extramuscular injection.

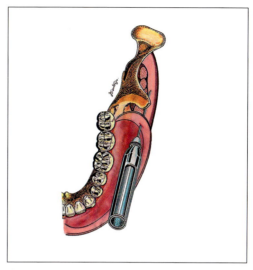

Fig 6-12 The intraoral injection of the masseter muscle area is shown. The anesthetic solution is injected external to muscle mass.

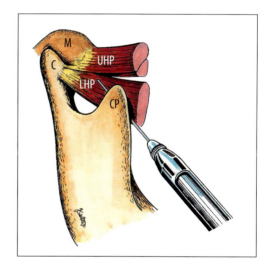

Fig 6-13 Intraoral injection of the external pterygoid muscle is shown. The anesthetic solution is injected external to the muscle. (UHP) Upper head of the lateral pterygoid muscle; (LHP) lower head of the lateral pterygoid muscle; (CP) coronoid process; (M) meniscus; (C) condyle.

the external fibers of the muscle (Fig 6-13). For this operation, the patient must be able to open the mouth to a reasonable extent.

A few complications of muscular injections have been noted clinically. The most significant one is lipothymia (fainting) of the patient. There is also the possibility of postoperative pain; in this case, the prescription of analgesics is recommended.

Temporomandibular joint injections

The infiltration of sclerosing, hyaluronidase, saline, steroid, and anesthetic solutions into the joints must be restricted to drastic circumstances under the continuous guidance of specialists. Side effects are almost inevitable, and the utilization of this invasive therapy may manifest outcomes beyond the control of the therapist. Intra-articular adhesions and structural degeneration may follow.

Arthrocentesis, arthroscopy, injections in the joint, and so on have been used consistently in the dental profession. The indications for these processes are supposed to be carefully considered, and advanced training is mandatory. Arthrocentesis, which can be characterized as puncture, aspiration, and even inflation of the joints, eventually followed by arthroscopic manipulations inside the joints to eliminate adhesions, is a technique that is well accepted by specialists in oral surgery lately.[2–5]

Iontophoresis

Iontophoresis[14] is the process in which, with the use of electrodes, ions of a given drug solution pass through the skin by passage of DC electrical current. There are several iontophoresis units on the market; most of them are activated with batteries. The negative (anode) electrode carries negative ions through the intact skin and the positive (cathode) electrode transmits the positive ions, using a very low current that is not perceived by the patient.

Many drugs can ionize into either positive or negative ions. For example, drugs with positive ionization may include epinephrine and lidocaine hydrochloride. Negative ionizing drugs may be represented by methyl prednisolone sodium succinate, dexamethasone sodium phosphate, and others.

There are some reports about the use of this process for the introduction of ionic corticosteroid into the temporomandibular joints to reverse inflammatory processes. Some authors even suggest the use of this process in combination with other forms of therapy for temporomandibular disorders[14]; however, its clinical use is relatively new and not all the aspects of its action are completely known.

EXTERNAL BIOFEEDBACK

Every living being manifests complex or simple internal organic mechanisms that provide a constant biofeedback loop to regulate biologic functions. With the recent development of some instruments, medical science has been able to develop external biofeedback strategies to increase interest in its use.[15–18]

This method is intended to promote homeostasis of selected physiologic functions. External biofeedback is a therapeutic technique in which patients learn how to gain control over their own physiologic functions through autogenous control. In the past, this approach was used in medicine as a diagnostic aid. However, lately there have been attempts to introduce this procedure for treatment of different forms of dysfunction.

Several modes of external biofeedback exist. One form, electroencephalographic biofeedback, is applied in psychotherapy, concentration, relaxation, and treatment of insomnia.

Another modality is galvanic skin resistance biofeedback. Emotional states, which are known to produce changes in sweat gland activity, altering the electrical resistance of the skin, can be detected by biofeedback instrumentation. This modality of treatment is used in psychotherapy as a demonstration medium and to promote imagery creation.

Another mode is temperature control biofeedback, which is distinctively applied to the extremities of the body. This kind of treatment has been used for circulatory problems such as migraine headaches and Raynaud disease.

The most commonly used modality is electromyographic biofeedback. Muscular activity can be successfully detected with the use of electromyography. The patient is connected to a special galvanometer capable of displaying the electrical activity of motor units in a given muscle. The instrument emits some form of audio and/or visual signals, making the patient aware of the muscular activity. This kind of muscle perception can familiarize patients with their internal physiologic processes, helping them to control the firing of muscle motor units. Because some emotional states may be connected with muscular hyperactivity, this type of therapy uses sessions of relaxation training to control muscle contraction. Recently, audible electromyographic biofeedback was introduced in dentistry for treatment of masticatory system disorders and has been shown to be a productive adjuvant.[16–18]

Naturally, training in electromyographic biofeedback must be appropriate for the patient's problem. Symptoms of TMD may be the result of causes other than muscular hyperactivity, such as tension headaches.

Relaxation training

Training sessions must be based, at the very beginning, on an informal and implicit contract between patient and therapist. This contract should state that:

- The reason for going through the procedure lies in the opportunity to experience the pleasurable feelings of relaxation.
- No particular long-range positive results are implied.
- No serious complications are expected.
- It is necessary to practice the relaxation procedures at home, twice a day.

Experience dictates that weekly appointments work well for relaxation training. Each session must have a duration of at least 30 minutes.

A reasonable gain in learning to relax the jaw muscles by use of audible electromyographic biofeedback may be expected to progress for at least 1 month. Later the patient will be able to relax by himself or herself using imagery strategies learned during the training sessions.

REFERENCES

1. Asahina I. Mandible bone regeneration using bone morphogenetic protein. Bull Kanagawa Dent Coll 2005;33:21–23.
2. Gangarosa LP, Mahan PE. Pharmacological management of temporomandibular joint muscle pain dysfunction syndrome. Ear Nose Throat J 1982;61:30–41.
3. Neidle EA, Yagiela JA. Pharmacology and Therapeutics for Dentistry, ed 3. St Louis: Mosby, 1989.
4. Phero JC. Pharmacotherapy for chronic facial pain. Dent Clin North Am 1984;28:471–491.
5. Ready LB, Brody MC. Drug problems in chronic pain patients. Anesthesiol Rev 1979;6:28–31.
6. Sherman M. A primer on use of hot and cold therapy. US Pharmacist Postgrad Pharm 1987;12:82–92.
7. Au AR, Klineberg IJ. Isokinetic exercise management of temporomandibular joint clicking in young adults. J Prosthet Dent 1983;70:33–38.
8. Stanko JR. A review of oral skeletal muscle relaxants for the craniomandibular disorder practitioner. Cranio 1990;8:234–243.
9. Mohl ND, Ohrbach RK, Crow HC, Gross AJ. Devices for the diagnosis and treatment of temporomandibular disorders. 3. Thermography, ultrasound, electrical stimulation and electromyographic biofeedback. J Prosthet Dent 1990;63:472–477.
10. Zwijnenburg AJ, Kroon GW, Verbeeten B Jr, Naeije M. Jaw movement responses to electrical stimulation of different parts of the human temporalis muscle. J Dent Res 1996;75:1798–1803.
11. Wessberg GA, Carroll WL, Dinham R, Wolford LM. Transcutaneous electrical stimulation as an adjunct in the management of myofascial pain dysfunction syndrome. J Prosthet Dent 1981;45:307–314.
12. Fordyce WE. On opioids and treatment targets. Am Pain Soc Bull 1991;1:1–34.
13. Turk DC, Zaki HS, Rudy TE. Effects of intraoral appliance and biofeedback/stress management alone and in combination in treating pain and depression in patients with temporomandibular disorders. J Prosthet Dent 1993;70:158–164.
14. Lark MR, Gangarosa LP. Iontophoresis: An effective modality for the treatment of inflammatory disorders of the temporomandibular joint and myofascial pain. Cranio 1990;8:108–119.
15. Basmajian JV. Biofeedback: Principles and Practice for Clinicians, ed 3. Baltimore: Williams & Wilkins, 1989:390.
16. Diamond S, Epstein MF. Biofeedback for headache. Biofeedback 1982;72:241–249.
17. Gaarner KR, Montgomery PS. Clinical Biofeedback: A Procedure Manual. Baltimore: Williams & Wilkins, 1977.
18. Nuechterlein KH, Holroyd JC. Biofeedback in the treatment of tension headache. Arch Gen Psychiatry 1980;37:866–873.

GEOMETRIC DETERMINANTS FOR FUNCTIONAL RESTORATIONS

7

Dental practitioners must control all aspects of their work. This is especially important with esthetic restorations, whether they are made directly in the patient's mouth or indirectly on mounted dies. All portions of dental crowns (anterior and posterior teeth) are shaped using carving procedures. This is especially important for occlusal surfaces. The traditional dental school curriculum of dental anatomy and functional occlusion concentrates on wax replacement of tooth structures. However, because of the characteristic format of these courses, little experience is gained in carving resin restoration patterns, specifically with rotary instruments, because these procedures are carried out after the final setting of the material.

In addition, with new esthetic materials that are placed directly in the patient's mouth, there is always the need:

- To perfect the axial contour of anterior crowns, with special emphasis on labial surfaces.
- To perfect the axial contour of posterior crown restorations for proper function and to avoid further problems (Figs 7-1 to 7-3). Reproduction of the correct labial or buccal flare of the embrasures is one of the best ways to preserve gingival health (Fig 7-4).
- To maintain the stability of the masticatory system with the correct contour of the occlusal surfaces of posterior teeth. Cuspal heights and the angle of cuspal inclines are critical parameters to establish during dental reconstructions.

Dental patients, depending on their age, degree of masticatory function, and characteristics of mandibular movements, present cusps with different angles and heights. For example, Fig 7-5 shows level curves obtained from two different types of occlusal reconstruction for the same subject. Depending on the different settings of the articulator used, the reconstructed maxillary first molars presented the same anatomic features but had different cuspal incline angulation and heights.

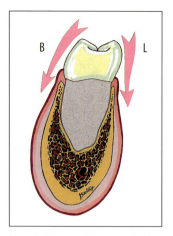

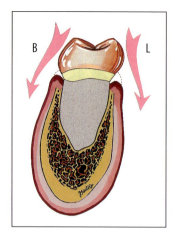

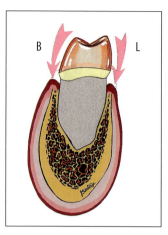

Fig 7-1 Normal axial contour of a dental crown and normal function, including proper adaptation to the free gingiva, stimulation and protection of the free gingival margin during chewing, and allowance for proper oral hygiene. *Arrows* indicate food flow. (B) Buccal; (L) lingual.

Fig 7-2 Excessive axial contour of a dental crown. Associated problems include unfavorable physiological stimulation with chewing, increased tonicity of the free gingiva and tendency for gingival recession, and impairment of oral hygiene measures leading to increased plaque retention. *Arrows* indicate food flow. (B) Buccal; (L) lingual.

Fig 7-3 Deficient axial contour of a dental crown. Associated problems include possible trauma to the free gingiva, increased food impaction, possible local inflammation and gingival recession, and reduced tonicity of the free gingiva. *Arrows* indicate food flow. (B) Buccal; (L) lingual.

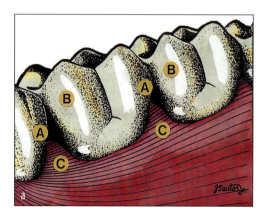

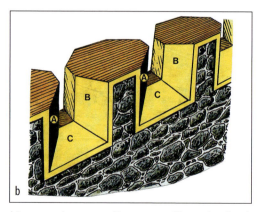

Fig 7-4 Anatomic concept of dental embrasures. The letters A, B, and C represent the corresponding structure of line angles of tooth crowns and gingival papilla *(a)*, as compared to the parts of a fortification *(b)*.

Based on preliminary observation of the geometric characteristics of groups of teeth, the objective of this chapter is to provide suggestions for the reader to define planar representation of these structures. This knowledge is crucial to the development of successful functional restorations, which will be illustrated in the second part of the chapter.

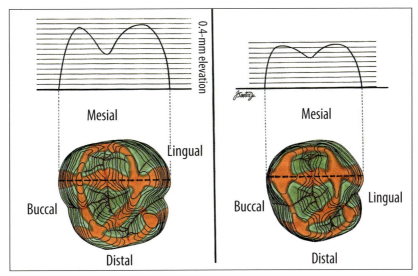

Fig 7-5 Level curves obtained from two different types of reconstruction for the same subject. Both maxillary first molars, although presenting the same anatomic features, have different cuspal inclines and heights.

GEOMETRIC REPRESENTATION OF ANTERIOR TEETH

The detailed observation of any tooth crown will disclose some interesting geometric aspects pertaining to lines and planes (Fig 7-6):

- Lines that can be defined along the long axis of the crowns represent axial contours and delineate lobes (Fig 7-7) and ridges. These lines delimit the greatest height of contour on the labial, buccal, lingual, incisal, occlusal, mesial, and distal aspects of the tooth (Fig 7-8).
- Lines that delineate the incisal or occlusal view of dental units represent the periphery of anterior and posterior crowns, which is called the *equator* of the tooth. Instead of being a straight line, as seen on the circumference of a sphere, it is a wavy line along the cervical, lingual, and interproximal heights of contour (Fig 7-9).
- Planes and inclines constitute the anatomic features of different crown elements, such as all external surfaces, line angles, cuspal inclines, and fossae (Figs 7-10 and 7-11).

These descriptions will exemplify the characteristics of the groups of teeth that can be used for single- or multiple-tooth reconstructions.

159

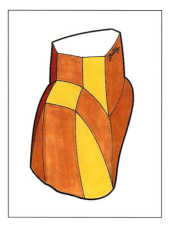

Fig 7-6 Planar representation of a maxillary central incisor.

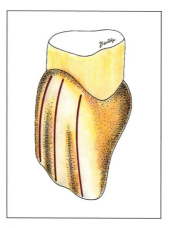

Fig 7-7 Lines defined along the long axis of the crown of a maxillary central incisor, representing axial contours and delineating lobes.

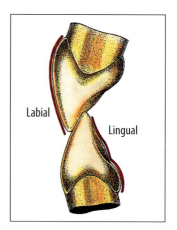

Fig 7-8 Outlines of the height of contour on the labial and lingual aspects of two opposing canines.

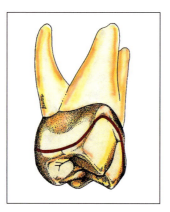

Fig 7-9 Outlines of the circumference of a maxillary molar, which is known as the *equator* of the tooth.

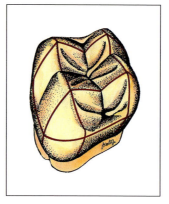

Fig 7-10 Different planes of a crown delineated by continuous lines, which follow the heights of contour. Those lines may represent the framework of the crown.

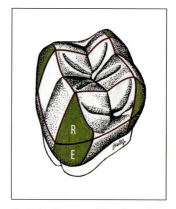

Fig 7-11 Retentive (R) and expulsive (E) portions of a molar, delimited by the outlines of the heights of contour of the crown.

Incisors

With different proportions, all incisors approximate the shape of a spatula. When the tooth is contoured, it is important to appreciate the position of the height of the axial contour on the labial and lingual areas. On these areas, the heights of contour are very close to cervical aspects of the crown and, in the majority of cases, present difficulties with the finish line of cavity preparations placed at the level of

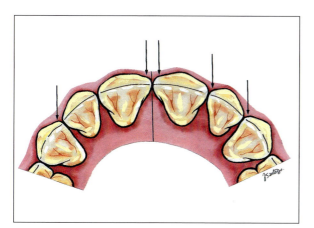

Fig 7-12 Line angles *(arrows)*, one of the most important features defining the labial surface of anterior teeth.

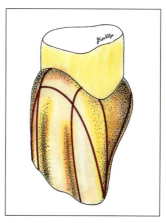

Fig 7-13 Line angles and other features of anterior teeth, delimited by the outlines of the heights of contour of the crown.

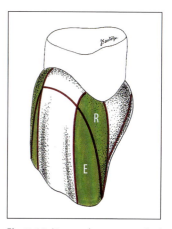

Fig 7-14 Line angles, composed of retentive (R) and expulsive (E) portions.

Fig 7-15 Developmental grooves *(red lines)*, common features on the labial surface of anterior teeth.

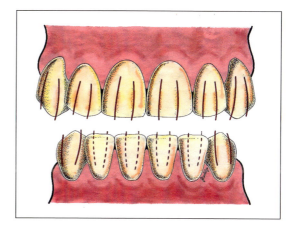

the gingival margin. However, the most critical aspect to obtaining proper proportion of the crowns is related to line angles (Fig 7-12). The natural appearance of these crowns can be easily ruined if the line angles encroach on labial embrasures.

Figures 7-13 and 7-14 depict a maxillary central incisor. Each line angle is composed of two small areas divided by the equator of the crown. One area (expulsive) is oriented incisally and the contiguous one (retentive) is oriented cervically. When forming line angles, the clinician must keep these aspects in mind to produce properly rounded corners of the crown.

During the finishing procedure for maxillary incisors, shallow depressions (developmental grooves) should be added to the labial surface (Fig 7-15). These grooves will vary the reflection of light, making the surface appear more natural.

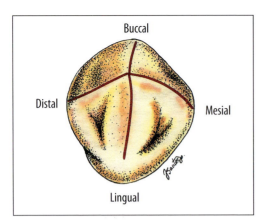

Fig 7-16 Pyramidal aspect of a canine when viewed from the incisal edge.

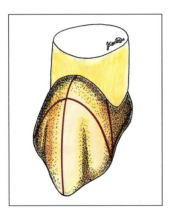

Fig 7-17 Outlines of the heights of contour and the equator of a canine.

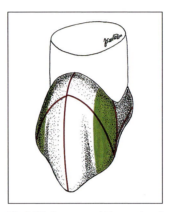

Fig 7-18 *(green areas)* Line angles of the crown of a canine, which is delimited by the outlines of the axial contours.

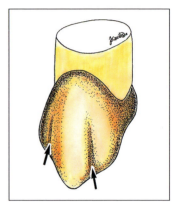

Fig 7-19 Developmental grooves *(arrows)* on each side of the central lobe on the labial surface of a canine.

Canines

Although the canine is not included among the posterior teeth, it can be viewed as a single-cusp tooth, which is why it is also called a *cuspid*. The crown has a pyramidal shape (Fig 7-16). The incisal edge of the tooth is composed of two ridges, and the vertex of the pyramid coincides with the cusp tip. The third ridge defines the labial central lobe, and the last ridge defines the lingual lobe.

All line angles of this tooth are divided by the equators of the crown (Figs 7-17 and 7-18).

It is important to add all the characteristic features of the labial surface (such as developmental grooves) when esthetic restoration of a canine is finished; this will enhance the natural appearance of the crown (Fig 7-19).

Fig 7-20 Planar representation of the occlusal view of two opposing quadrants of the left side.

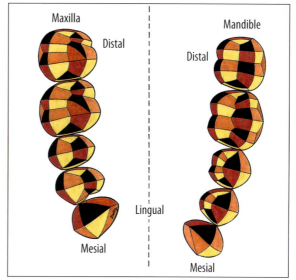

GEOMETRIC REPRESENTATION OF OCCLUSAL SURFACES

Familiarity with the morphologic aspects of the occlusal surface of the teeth enables the dental practitioner to understand the functional balance of masticatory processes and to plan the reconstruction of the whole or part of the masticatory apparatus. This balance may be better understood when the details of occlusal surfaces are observed, especially when those elements are directly involved with mastication.

The anatomy of occlusal surfaces involved in mastication invariably presents spatial orientations, which may indicate the type of functional activity developed during the chewing of the food. To an attentive observer, the planar characteristics of this spatial formation are inescapable. Objective analysis of the geometric occlusal surfaces of posterior teeth is illustrated according to dynamic or functional patterns (planar representation). For example, Fig 7-20 shows an occlusal view of the left-side maxillary and mandibular quadrants according to geometric features. In these geometric representations, inclines were made visible to suggest their gliding directions on chewing surfaces. Customarily, gliding movements between opposing occlusal surfaces are produced during functional (or even sometimes parafunctional) grinding.

Based on the concept that the morphology of the teeth represents an important role in masticatory function, attention to geometric patterns may serve as a useful guide in the creation of an occlusal configuration capable of preserving proper function and stability of the system. Mandibular kinematics is mostly governed by tooth morphology, neuromuscular control, masticatory muscles, and temporomandibular joints. These essential components of the masticatory apparatus interplay harmoniously in normal maxillomandibular relationships, especially at the centric position and during eccentric displacements of the jaw.

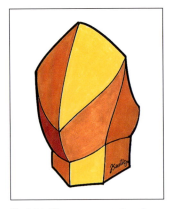

Fig 7-21 Planar representation of a canine crown (tooth with just one cusp).

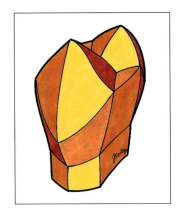

Fig 7-22 Planar representation of a premolar crown (tooth with two cusps).

Occlusal prematurities prevent stable intercuspation. These interferences to smooth functional movements during mastication are distortions that may be found in some occlusal schemes, either from natural variations or from poor dentistry. Sometimes, these morphologic changes of the dentition deleteriously influence and alter the equilibrium of the whole masticatory system.

It is possible to define some geometric parameters to describe the occlusal surface of posterior teeth. Primarily, these surfaces are composed of functional units called *cusps*. A single cusp can be geometrically depicted as a four-sided pyramid (Fig 7-21).

Premolars

The majority of premolars may be geometrically represented by a grouping of two cusps, the reason why they are also called *bicuspids* (Fig 7-22), and eventually three cusps. A geometric representation of the occlusal surface of teeth depicts two four-sided pyramids of different sizes that are linked together, side by side. Their respective bases sit on the same horizontal plane. These pyramids are oriented in such a way that one of the ridges of the first is roughly in the same alignment with a ridge of the second pyramid. These ridges correspond to triangular ridges of the occlusal surface of the crown. Starting from each side of the vertex of each pyramid, in the mesiodistal direction, it is possible to detect the appearance of corresponding cusp arms. The central buccal and lingual lobes are represented by the external ridges of the pyramids. Finally, the mesial and distal triangular fossae are delineated by triangular facets.

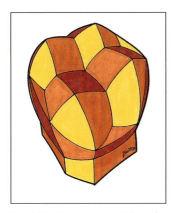

Fig 7-23 Planar representation of a mandibular second molar (tooth with four cusps).

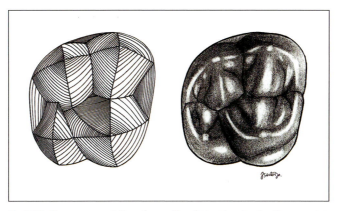

Fig 7-24 Planar representation of a maxillary first molar, showing the geometric characteristics of four pyramids linked side by side as compared to the anatomic crown. The mesiolingual cusp is represented as a five-sided pyramid.

Molars

Molars are geometrically illustrated as teeth with four or more cusps (Fig 7-23). Thus, the occlusal surfaces of molars with four cusps are composed of the same number of different sized, four-sided pyramids resting on the same horizontal plane and linked side by side at the level of two of the cuspal ridges of each one. This disposition represents the formation of mandibular second molars. Mandibular first molars are characterized by five pyramids, three of them located on the buccal side. Maxillary molars are also composed of four pyramids, but for the sake of didactic description, the mesiolingual cusp may be symbolized as a five-sided pyramid instead (Fig 7-24). In all examples, the central occlusal fossa of each crown is formed when two groups of pyramids are connected.

FUNCTIONAL DIRECT SINGLE RESTORATIONS

As observed previously, single-tooth carving is not a very difficult process when all geometric principles are rigorously followed. After the geometric model is ascertained, the final anatomic features can be carved to perfect the particular characteristics inherent to a given tooth.

When working directly in the patient's mouth, the clinician requires a more elaborate process. Besides simulating anatomic characteristics, the restoration that is carved must comply with its functional role in the dental arch. The anatomic reproduction of a tooth crown should be compatible with other features of teeth in the same or opposing arches, including esthetics; cross-arch symmetry; interproximal contacts and relations; embrasures; interocclusal relationships; and cervical contours (Fig 7-25).

When using a technique based on functionally generated paths formed by bite imprinting (commonly known as the *chew-in technique*), the clinician must assume that the morphologic characteristics of opposing teeth are satisfactory. If opposing teeth are absent, other morphologic information must be considered, such as contiguity with teeth in the same arch (Fig 7-26); symmetry with the corresponding crown on the other side of the arch; and the occlusal plane.

When the restoration is being fabricated directly in the patient's mouth, the choice of this kind of procedure is primarily associated with extensive loss of occlusal relationships. The technique presented in this chapter is for crown patterns for cast restorations as well as for bonded resin restorations. However, bonded resin restorations should be placed with rubber dam isolation, making direct carving in the patient's mouth very difficult. Also, in this case, "slump" of flow is a problem during buildup of prepolymerized cuspal elevations.

A restorative process carried out directly in the dental arch using casts mounted on a semiadjustable articulator will be described. This discussion will not concentrate on the technique for or type of cavity preparations. The objective is to describe how to reproduce patterns of interocclusal relationships through carving.

Irrespective of the type of cavity preparation, if cusps are supposed to be replaced through occlusal reconstruction, it is necessary to provide interocclusal clearance for the restorative material. This clearance must have an even thickness of at least 2 mm in relation to opposing teeth (Fig 7-27). Further reduction of the occlusal surface of one or more teeth will provide space for insertion of material for carving.

Insertion of material

Tooth-colored, unpolymerized resin composite or autopolymerizing acrylic resin is adapted to the simulated cavity preparation (full crown or box preparation). An incremental cone is recommended for placement of light-curing resin composites, especially where the thickness of the material is more than 2 mm. The material may present a slight overflow in relation to the occlusal surfaces of adjacent teeth. The opposing teeth are made to touch firmly in maximum intercuspation (Fig 7-28). Adjacent and opposing teeth involved in this procedure should be lubricated. It should be confirmed that the opposing crown is producing indentations in the soft material. Any excess material can be easily removed when it is still uncured.

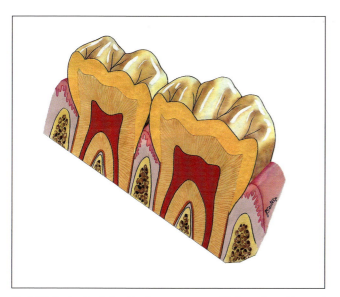

Fig 7-25 Anatomic relationships between two mandibular molars with regard to marginal ridges, buccal cusp tips, interproximal space, mesiodistal occlusal developmental grooves, gingival space, and supporting structures.

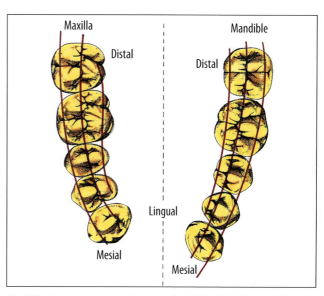

Fig 7-26 Continuity of anatomic features (mesiodistal developmental grooves, buccal cusp tips, and lingual cusp tips) of occlusal surfaces, from one tooth to another, as observed on two opposing dental quadrants of the left side.

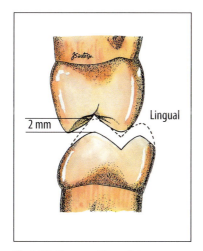

Fig 7-27 Clearance of 2 mm between opposing teeth to create space for carving.

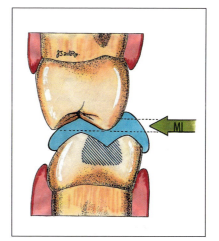

Fig 7-28 Soft material *(blue area)* in position and opposing teeth closed in maximum intercuspation (MI).

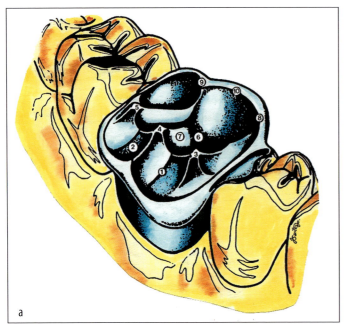

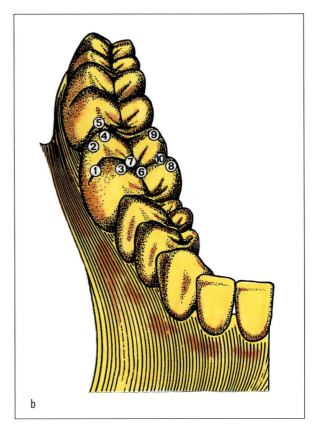

Fig 7-29 Usual appearance of the indentations on the soft material (*a*), produced by an opposing tooth (*b*). The numbers 1 to 10 represent corresponding anatomic features of the indentation and the intact crown. (1 and 2) Location of future buccal grooves between the developmental lobes of the mesiobuccal, distobuccal, and distal cusps; (3, 4, and 5) further location of buccal supporting cusps, although very pointed at this time; (6) support of opposing cusp; (7) one of the occlusal inclines of the distobuccal cusp—other inclines are also distinguishable; (8 and 9) future position of the cusp tips of lingual nonsupporting cusps; (10) orientation of the lingual groove.

Reading the occlusal imprints

After the material has set, the articulator is opened to disclude the teeth and permit a reading of the indentations on the resin. Figure 7-29 shows impressions produced by the maxillary right first molar on the soft material that was used to replace the occlusal surface of the opposing mandibular right first molar.

The restoration is now cured, according to the manufacturer's recommendation, with a light wand or another appropriate source of visible light.

The patient's and clinician's eyes must be protected with filters.

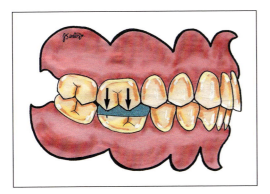

Fig 7-30 Buccal grooves *(arrows)* on the mandibular crown in relation to the maxillary molar. Buccal view.

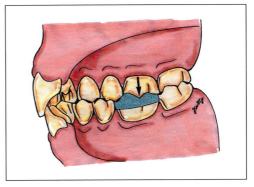

Fig 7-31 Orientation of the lingual groove *(arrow)* of the mandibular crown in relation to the maxillary molar. Lingual view.

Carving the occlusal restoration

If indentations are well produced, the carving of the occlusal surface with rotary instruments is not supposed to be a very complicated task. Based on geometric principles used for single-unit carving, the following steps are performed for carving of restorations on articulated casts.

First, the excess resin that remains on the buccal and/or lingual sides of the crown is removed. It is necessary to proceed carefully to avoid overreduction. At this stage, buccal and lingual developmental lobes and grooves are created, according to the guidance provided by the height of contour of adjacent teeth and opposing crowns (Figs 7-30 and 7-31). It is important to define the size of embrasures by carving out the excess material at the level of the line angles (see Fig 7-11).

Next, the position of the marginal ridges is adjusted. Any overhang of material must be eliminated, but care must be taken to avoid damaging the occlusal surface.

Occlusal cuspal inclines are now defined with small, rotary-mounted points in accordance with the geometric pattern for the crown being carved. The geometric orientation of these inclines must be clearly defined as the sides of the pyramids. These inclines are limited by the mesiodistal and buccolingual grooves of the occlusal surface. The carving process may be carried out with high-speed burs.

Once the occlusal surface has been defined, all sharp edges are rounded. Rotary instruments are used again to work directly on ridges and cusp tips. Secondary anatomy, secondary grooves, or other anatomic details of the occlusal surface are added at this time. Secondary grooves are shallow depressions on the surface of each incline and are limited by the triangular ridges of each cusp. All occlusal details should present a continuity of the features shown by adjacent teeth. For example, the alignment of mesial and lingual cusp tips, as well as

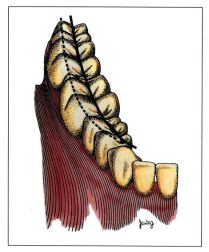

Fig 7-32 Continuity of buccal cusp tips *(dotted line)* and central grooves *(solid line)* in a mandibular right quadrant.

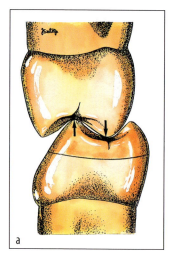
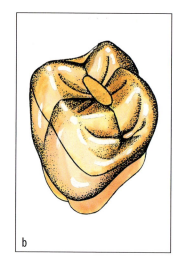

Fig 7-33 Adjustment for freedom in centric *(a)* for all ranges of movements. The result will be the creation of a flat platform *(b)* for the opposing cusp.

mesiodistal grooves, represents a practically continuous line from tooth to tooth in the same arch (Fig 7-32).

When carving is performed directly in the patient's mouth, functional chewing movements can be produced. This method is useful to check for premature contacts in the range between maximum intercuspation, centric relation, and eccentric interferences. The adjustment for freedom in centric (as explained in detail in chapter 8) can be produced for all ranges of movement; the result will be the generation of a flat platform for the opposing cusp (Fig 7-33).

Finally, the restoration is smoothed and finished. This task is carried out with the aid of finishing burs and points. The operator must pay attention to minute details. No small ripples should exist before final polishing is begun.

OCCLUSAL ADJUSTMENT OF THE ADULT NATURAL DENTITION

Occlusal adjustment encompasses the equilibration of the natural dentition through various approaches. There are many techniques for occlusal adjustment. All are equally effective when performed in compliance with the occlusal philosophical concepts on which they are based. Although many procedures may be applied for occlusal adjustment (from simple "spot grinding" to complex orthognathic surgery), this chapter describes one technique for occlusal adjustment: selective grinding according to the concept of freedom in centric.

Freedom-in-centric adjustment of the natural dentition may be accomplished by any professional without the need for expensive instrumentation and is easily learned. Occlusal adjustment represents a comprehensive procedure in which no harm will be imposed on the masticatory system. The creation of a flat area on the depth of the fossa is compatible with basic principles related to the freedom-in-centric concept and maintains chewing loads along the longitudinal axis of the teeth. No deficient chewing will result from this adjustment.

Freedom-in-centric adjustment, according to its followers, is an open-ended concept that has no place for dogmatists. Frequently, when an occlusal adjustment according to freedom-in-centric principles is being planned, different decisions are required. For example, sometimes it is not possible to plan for this adjustment in the range between centric relation and centric occlusion when:

- An extensive slide in centric is detected because of the anterior displacement of the discs in the joints.
- There is a possibility that cusp tips would be ground, probably as a result of the aforementioned condition or because of arch discrepancies.
- Centric occlusion and centric relation are coincident positions.
- There is an occasional inability to properly manipulate the mandible in centric relation because of, for example, the presence of some form of muscle splinting.

The first three situations mentioned may represent serious contraindications to centric adjustment, but will never preclude the need for occlusal adjustment of other mandibular eccentric positions. Any adjustment just comprising eccentric

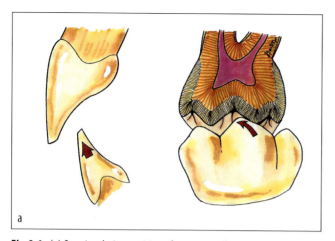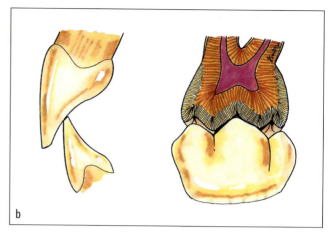

Fig 8-1 *(a)* Centric relation position of segments of opposing arches. *(arrows)* Direction of the slide. *(b)* Maximum intercuspation contact at the molars and anterior teeth.

movements of the mandible may be considered a limited adjustment. The last condition, however, may represent a predicament when comprehensive occlusal adjustment is planned. No occlusal adjustment procedure should be started in the presence of muscle splinting. Patients who require comprehensive occlusal adjustment may be initially subjected to bite splint therapy.

GOALS

Improvement of masticatory function

The clinician may improve the masticatory function of patients by applying the freedom-in-centric adjustment, irrespective of the craniomandibular status. However, the absence of pathologic signs and symptoms in the masticatory apparatus represents a consequential factor for occlusal assessment. A slide in centric may reveal the presence of unstable maxillomandibular relationships in the range between maximum intercuspation and centric relation, when teeth are clenched (Fig 8-1). Freedom-in-centric adjustment of the dentition may be considered a therapeutic procedure as part of the solution for occlusal and masticatory problems.

In addition, the creation of three-dimensional freedom at the level of interocclusal relationships may prevent contact interferences during eccentric mandibular movements (Fig 8-2). It has been accepted that interferences may lead to restricted chewing

Fig 8-2 Type of adjustment commonly performed on posterior teeth, which complies with the principles of freedom in centric. A platform is produced at the depth of the fossa, providing a three-dimensional seating area for the opposing cusp. The dotted lines starting from the center of the platform show the anterior-posterior (A-P) extension of the adjustment as well as the right-left extension (R-L). The direction of the occlusal force (F) is parallel to the long axis of the tooth. The range of this adjustment should produce long-term stability in maximum intercuspation, even during the constant functional wear of the dentition. In the vertical direction, the centric adjustment is limited by the vertical dimension of occlusion. *Red dots* represent centric occlusion contact.

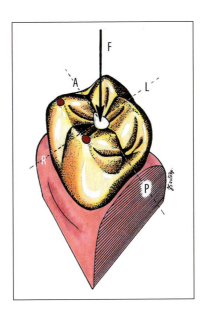

patterns of movement. The presence of parafunction and interferences may aggravate bruxism and precipitate dysfunction of the masticatory system.[1]

Alleviation of bruxism

Patients with bruxism usually grind their teeth in centric relation during sleep and may be subjected to continuous "empty swallowing." Any prematurity at the level of centric relation is prone to generate unconscious grinding and consequent hyperactivity of masticatory muscles. Consequently, prematurities in centric relation may be regarded not as restrictive but rather as a powerful stimulus to perpetuate bruxism.[1–5] The elimination of prematurities in centric relation will not guarantee the resolution of bruxism; however, it is a stratagem to stabilize interocclusal relationships for better distribution of forces during clenching.

Simplification of articulator use

From a technical point of view, an occlusal adjustment done according to the principles of freedom in centric is capable of helping the operator to properly mount articulators when extensive restorative procedures are necessary. Articulators are made for remounting, and there is no way to provide consistent remounting if the casts are not related on the instrument according to centric relation position. Therefore, if the mandible is manipulated into reproducible centric relation and this position is captured with an occlusal record, no predicaments will be expected during rehabilitation procedures. In this case, the reconstruction will start in centric relation and then proceed to other positions.

INDICATIONS

The application of the knowledge of occlusion in everyday dentistry must be consistent, especially when the clinician is performing diverse forms of occlusal therapy. From the simple approach of spot grinding to comprehensive rehabilitation, when exercising occlusal equilibration the operator must have a clear idea about its principles and indications. Dental professionals must be aware that once procedures for adjustment are started, there is no way to reverse the situation. The adjustment of the dentition is an invasive procedure that is considered irreversible and must be well planned in advance.

Clinical conditions that demand careful assessment of occlusal relationships must define which variety of treatment may be carried out to maintain or improve the stability of the masticatory system. Among others, the following clinical situations may involve procedures for occlusal equilibration.

Occlusal trauma

The need for adjustment because of occlusal trauma must be chiefly based on the diagnosis of the problem, rather than on the presence of occlusal prematurities and interferences, which in some cases do not bear any significance. However, if treatment is planned, occlusal adjustment should be the treatment of choice in the presence of signs and/or symptoms of occlusal trauma.

Limited movements of the mandible

Some patients develop limited movement to avoid pain or for chewing convenience. In the majority of cases, the presence of premature contacts in centric positions and occlusal interferences in eccentric movements (working, balancing, and protrusive movements as well as any range between these movements) is the result of the collapse of the occlusion. This collapse may be caused by:

- Loss of vertical dimension
- Absence of teeth
- Faulty restorative and corrective procedures (which may include orthodontics, orthopedic manipulations, restorative dentistry, surgery, intraoral appliances, prosthodontics, etc)
- Bruxism and parafunctional habits[1-5]
- Increased tooth mobility and loss of periodontal support[6]
- Caries
- Faulty occlusal adjustment

An occlusal adjustment in these cases may improve the patient's comfort and function. However, in some clinical situations, it has limited influence on the results of the treatment.[1,4,5]

Bruxism and disorders of the masticatory system

The idea that occlusal adjustment is capable of curing bruxism or any dysfunction of the masticatory system has not been totally proved. However, occlusal adjustment may help to improve the function and stability of the masticatory apparatus.[1,4,5]

After orthodontics, orthognathic surgery, and other forms of surgical correction

There are some recommendations for the prescription of an occlusal adjustment after surgery and/or orthodontics to provide stability and even to prevent relapse after treatment.[7] The objective is improvement of function, because some corrections accomplished through surgery or tooth movements may produce occlusal instability. Eventually, occlusal equilibration may represent the only acceptable alternative to correct instability at the level of the dentition.

Before restorative dentistry

Prior to any kind of extensive restorative procedure, occlusal adjustment may define a serviceable baseline, as a starting point for restorations; however, the patient must be free of dysfunctional signs and/or symptoms in the masticatory system.

During periodontal therapy

The effect of occlusal adjustment on periodontal therapy was evaluated during a 2-year clinical study. The results demonstrated that patients who received occlusal adjustment had a significantly greater gain of clinical periodontal attachment than did the group who only received independent modalities of periodontal treatment and no adjustment.[6] Although the results of this study may be questioned, it is evident that occlusal adjustment must deserve special consideration as an adjunct to periodontal treatment for the retention of teeth.

OCCLUSAL ADJUSTMENT ON MOUNTED CASTS

Any experienced clinician should be able to undertake selective grinding of the natural dentition directly in the patient's mouth. However, it is always advisable to initiate the planning process in advance. It is good procedure to start the grinding on the patient's casts mounted on a semiadjustable articulator. It is also a good idea to paint the areas ground on the casts with a highlighting marker (for example, orange) to clarify the position and amount of tooth reduction.

The real advantage of these procedures lies in the fact that, after completion of the adjustment on casts, it will be easy for the professional to visualize the final results, to make final decisions, and to explain the subsequent intraoral treatment to the patient. The following sections describe procedures for occlusal adjustment carried out on mounted casts. The sequence presented is comprehensive and appropriate for achieving freedom in centric in the majority of circumstances.

When casts are mounted on a semiadjustable articulator with a centric relation bite record, there is a provision for slide in centric (ie, a range of movement between maximum intercuspation and centric relation). Casts properly mounted on the articulator should produce stable intercuspation (Fig 8-3). This condition represents the contact vertical dimension of the casts in maximum intercuspation. When the articulator is moved in maximum intercuspation:

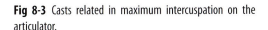

Fig 8-3 Casts related in maximum intercuspation on the articulator.

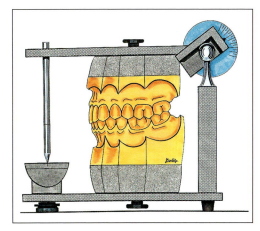

- The condylar spheres should not be resting against the posterior wall of the condylar housing, and there should be a small space between this ball and the posterior wall. This space roughly corresponds to the amount of displacement of the condyles in the joints from centric relation to maximum intercuspation.
- The incisal pin should be in contact with the center of its incisal table (Figs 8-4 and 8-5). There might be a slight deviation of the pin to one of the sides if the patient presents a lateral component of slide in centric (Fig 8-6 and 8-7).

If the articulator is moved again into centric relation, the condylar balls must rest against the posterior walls of their respective condylar housings. Therefore, there will be no more stable interocclusal contacts. The contact vertical dimension in centric relation is greater than maximum intercuspation. A sliding movement between centric relation and maximum intercuspation is evidence that the articulator is dislodging from an unstable position in centric relation to achieve stable intercuspal interdigitations (Fig 8-8).

For the articulator to be considered in centric relation:

- The condylar spheres must be centered, according to a common axis of rotation, in their respective condylar housings (Fig 8-8).
- The lower extremity of the incisal pin must be moved forward, and there must be no contact with the incisal table (see Figs 8-5 and 8-8). This characteristic represents the vertical, horizontal, and eventually lateral dimensions of the components of the slide in centric.

For better discernment of the spatial components of the slide, the incisal table must be kept flat during this procedure.

For eccentric movements, other settings are obtained and related to the condylar elements of the instrument. Thus, the use of a protrusive checkbite (and for

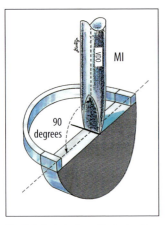

Fig 8-4 Incisal pin vertically touching (90 degrees) the center of the incisal table at intercuspal position (MI). The pin has been adjusted according to the vertical dimension of occlusion (VDO).

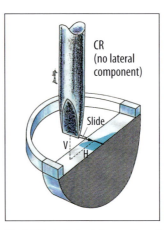

Fig 8-5 Incisal pin at the position of the articulator in centric relation (CR) without lateral deviation (no lateral component). The slide has vertical (V) and horizontal components (H).

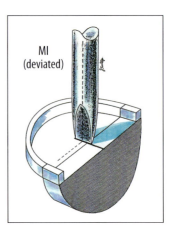

Fig 8-6 Incisal pin touching the incisal table in maximum intercuspation (MI) with deviation to one side.

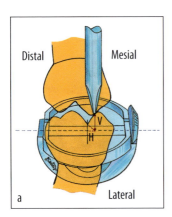

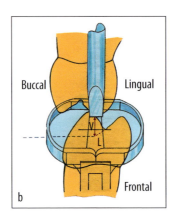

Fig 8-7 Lateral (a) and frontal (b) views of the incisal table and incisal pin when the articulator is moved in centric relation. A first centric relation contact is produced between two opposing right first molars. The incisal pin that is not touching the center of the table and the upper and anterior displacement of the incisal pin define the approximate extension of the slide in centric, which is long. The slide is eccentric and presents three components: vertical (V), horizontal (H), and lateral (L).

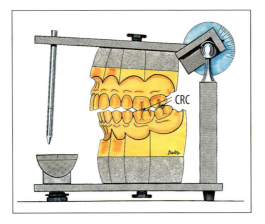

Fig 8-8 Casts mounted on the articulator now related in centric relation and showing occlusal contacts in that position (CRC).

Fig 8-9 Opposing arches of the left side will be used as an example for explanation of occlusal adjustment. The relationships of opposing teeth are detailed at the level of canines, premolars, and molars on both quadrants of the left side. *(red dots)* Centric stops; *(green dots)* centric relation contact; *(dotted lines)* centric position orientation of supporting cusps as they touch the corresponding opposing teeth. The red dots represent portions of the occlusal surface usually involved in maximum intercuspation and must be avoided during adjustment. The green marks represent centric relation prematurities and, conventionally, areas where the adjustment can be performed. (D) Distal; (M) mesial; (B) buccal; (L) lingual.

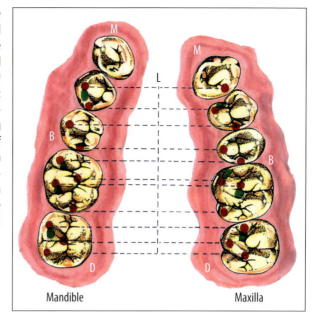

Mandible   Maxilla

some articulator models, lateral checkbites) allows setting of the horizontal condylar guidance and the Bennett angle.

When articulators are used, the setting of the Fischer angle on the instrument has limited significance to the concept of freedom in centric, as far as functional occlusion is concerned. If the Fischer angle is to be considered, its association with functional occlusion is represented by attainment or perpetuation of proficient canine guidance.

Occlusal analysis

Contacts in centric positions

Before making any judgment about where to adjust the occlusion, the clinician must survey tooth contact between opposing arches. As a starting point, the articulator is moved into centric relation. In most cases, it is possible for premature or first centric relation contacts to occur between supporting cusps of both arches (Fig 8-9). The expression *premature contact* implies that, when the instrument is guided into centric relation and opposing arches are contacting, it is essential to have just one first contact or a few centric relation unstable contacts. It is probable that not all teeth are going to be in contact in centric relation at this stage.

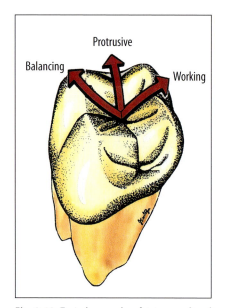

Fig 8-10 Typical example of intercuspal and eccentric relationships when a supporting cusp exits the opposing fossa. The paths of the opposing cusp moving away from centric position *(arrows)* in protrusive, balancing, and working movements are shown.

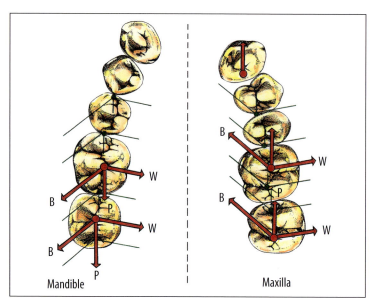

Fig 8-11 Direction of movement *(red arrows and green lines)* in protrusive (P), balancing (B), and working (W) movements.

Figure 8-9 defines the representation of opposing quadrants on the left side that will be used in the remainder of the chapter to explain details of tooth contacts and selective grinding. In the figure, centric relation contacts may be detected. Usually, the distal inclines of the supporting cusps of mandibular molars and premolars have a propensity to touch the mesial inclines of the supporting cusps of opposing maxillary posterior teeth.

Contacts in eccentric positions

Numerous interocclusal gliding motions are produced during excursive movements (Fig 8-10). Figure 8-11 demonstrates the associated trajectories developed by cusps exiting their respective fossae during balancing, working, and protrusive border movements of the mandible. These trajectories are comparable to a "dove's footprint" entering the mouth in the mandibular arch and leaving in the maxillary arch (Fig 8-12). Descriptions involving occlusal pathways are always based on the idea that supporting cusps are exiting opposing fossae (Fig 8-13).

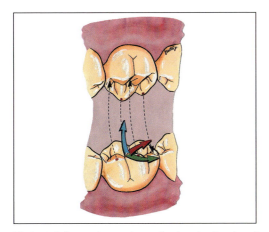

Fig 8-12 Left opposing quadrants showing the direction of movement *(blue, red, and green arrows)* of supporting cusps exiting the corresponding fossae. *Red dots* and *black arrows* represent the path of the mandibular supporting cusps entering a centric stop on the maxillary molar.

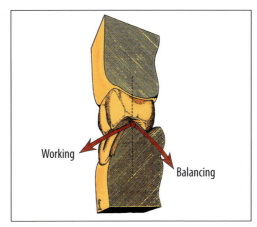

Fig 8-13 Movement of a mandibular supporting cusp exiting the fossa in working and balancing movements.

Balancing movement

Two opposing supporting cusps (lingual maxillary and buccal mandibular) have the potential for interference. In cases of crossbite, this relationship is not going to occur. Although they are used for artificial tooth mounting during denture construction, when they occur in the natural dentition balancing-side contacts may be considered balancing interferences or cross-arch balance. Figure 8-14 illustrates opposing quadrants on the left side displaying the inclines typically associated with balancing interferences.

Working movement

Total or partial group function (Fig 8-15) describes nonsupporting cusps that glide against supporting cusps. Usually, the buccal cusps of maxillary posterior teeth are involved in the working action against the buccal cusps of mandible posterior teeth. Nevertheless, it is considered working interference or cross-tooth balance when maxillary and mandibular cusps of posterior teeth on the lingual side restrict uniform working motions during mastication (Fig 8-16). This working relationship is not possible in cases of posterior crossbite. Figure 8-17 illustrates the inclines habitually involved in group function and working interference.

Protrusive movement

Nonsupporting cusps of maxillary posterior teeth may restrict the movement of mandibular supporting cusps. In the same fashion, nonsupporting cusps of mandibular teeth are possible interferences to supporting cusps of maxillary teeth. Figure 8-18 displays the inclines involved in these interferences. As applied to protrusive guidance, this type of guidance is mostly related to anterior teeth.

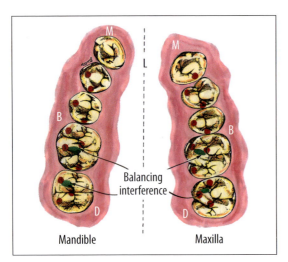

Fig 8-14 Involvement of the occlusal inclines and axial contours *(green dots)* during balancing movement in the left quadrants. *(red dots)* Centric stops; (D) distal; (M) mesial; (B) buccal; (L) lingual.

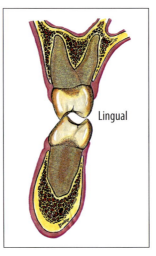

Fig 8-15 Molars in a working relationship during group function.

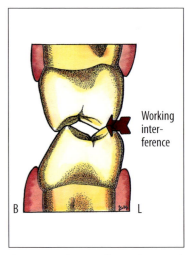

Fig 8-16 Working interference (cross-tooth balance). (B) Buccal; (L) lingual.

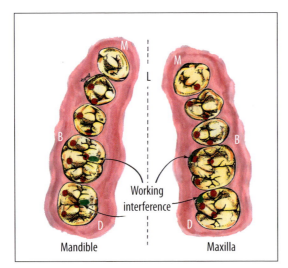

Fig 8-17 Occlusal inclines *(green dots)* that may contact in working movement in the left quadrants. Group function. *(red dots)* Centric stops; (D) distal; (M) mesial; (B) buccal; (L) lingual.

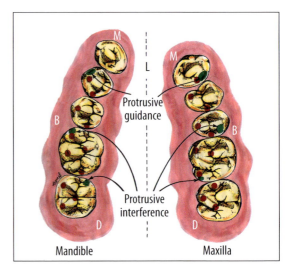

Fig 8-18 Occlusal cuspal inclines and axial contours *(green dots)* potentially involved in protrusive movement in the left quadrants. *(red dots)* Centric stops; (D) distal; (M) mesial; (B) buccal; (L) lingual.

Fig 8-19 Planar representation of occlusal contacts on inclines. Each color represents the occlusal contact for each maxillomandibular relationship: centric relation *(blue)*; balancing (cross-arch balance) *(red)*; canine guidance *(dark green)*; working guidance (group function) *(light green)*; working interference (cross-tooth balance) *(yellow)*; protrusive guidance *(orange)*; protrusive interference *(pink)*. (D) Distal; (M) mesial; (L) lingual.

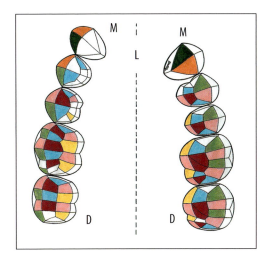

Preparatory decisions

Preparatory to any grinding procedure, the clinician must analyze the interocclusal relationships of the casts in all centric and eccentric movements. However, this protocol does not provide a sequence of steps to embody every minor decision to be made during an occlusal adjustment.

The observations described in this chapter will help to conceptualize the adjustment of occlusion, in the range between maximum intercuspation and centric relation as well as for eccentric movements. Based on these routines, it is possible to make decisions about where to grind when tooth contacts are analyzed.

Figure 8-19 presents a simplified planar representation of the occlusal surfaces of opposing left quadrants, where inclines were colored according to their functional relationships in the mouth. This scheme is useful to help guide decisions about where to grind in the majority of cases. During the sequence of analysis, it is advisable to start first in the centric positions and then proceed to the eccentric positions.

Centric positions

The concept of freedom in centric provides some guidelines for adjustment. These observations are very useful during the planning stages of an occlusal adjustment. The planning stages will help the operator to decide, before starting the grinding, whether or not the procedure would mutilate the dentition or if the relationship of the teeth is conducive to the attainment of stable interocclusal relationships.

Prematurities in centric relation

Although presenting plausible contacts in the maximum intercuspal position, casts placed in the centric relation position may reveal a great variety of first contact relationships at this level. In addition, the slide from centric relation to maximum intercuspation almost never occurs in a straightforward movement. Some reasons for this variation will be discussed in the following sections.

Configuration of the arches

Some patients have curvature incongruence between opposing arches. For example, a maxillary arch may present a triangular configuration and the mandibular arch may present an ovoid shape.

In other circumstances, when the mandible is manipulated in centric relation, the hinge axis of rotation in this position is not parallel to the horizontal transverse axis between condyles when teeth are in maximum intercuspation. Figure 8-20 demonstrates the variation of three hinge axes. In each case, variable centric slides can be detected between opposing supporting cusps when the teeth make first contact in centric relation. If the hinge axis is parallel to the intercondylar axis in maximum intercuspation, a straight slide may occur (see Fig 8-20b). If the hinge axis is not parallel, different degrees of lateral deviation of the jaw to one side can occur in centric relation (see Figs 8-20c and 8-20d).

Temporomandibular joint relationships

Patients may also exhibit a long slide (more than 2 mm) from centric relation to maximum intercuspation, probably because of some remodeling process within the joints or dysfunctional masticatory problems. In both circumstances, the presence of any incongruity between dental arches in this range of movement may be best assessed at the posterior teeth. When casts are properly mounted on an articulator with a centric relation occlusal record, the articulator will be able to capture the patient's exact centric relation first contacts.

Selection of areas to grind

To determine which areas to grind, the operator must first observe the occlusal portion of the supporting cusps of posterior teeth when visualizing areas of the occlusal tables. In Figs 8-20 and 8-21, to provide better clarity, these areas were individually colored:

- When the first centric relation contact between supporting cusps falls within the limits of the central groove of opposing teeth (*green areas*), this is an indication that the patient has a short, straightforward slide from centric relation to maximum intercuspation. Occlusal adjustment in this case should not cause complications as far stability is concerned.
- When the first centric relation contact relationship falls at the level of the cuspal inclines (*yellow areas*), the conditions are normal for the natural dentition, and the only consideration is the contact in centric relation. In this case, the centric

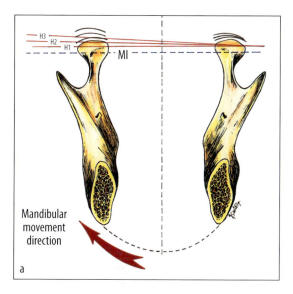

Mandibular movement direction

a

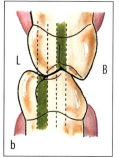

b

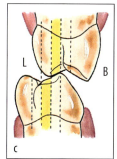

c

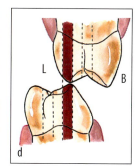

d

Fig 8-20 *(a)* Different transverse hinge axes in centric relation (H1, H2, and H3) as compared to the transverse axis in maximum intercuspation (MI). *(b to d)* Occlusal contact relationships in centric relation with different hinge axes: *(b)* H1 straight slide; *(c)* H2 lateral centric relation deviation; *(d)* H3 excessive deviation. (B) Buccal; (L) lingual.

Fig 8-21 The green, yellow and red areas represent possible occlusal relationships of the posterior teeth when the mandible is in centric relation. *Black dots* represent cuspal areas of contact in centric occlusion; *white dots* represent areas of centric occlusion contact on opposing teeth.

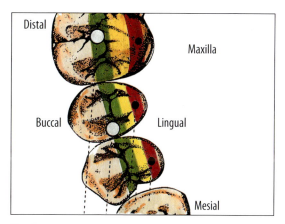

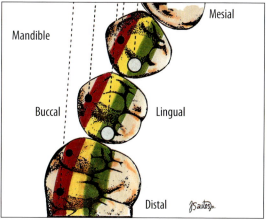

occlusal adjustment may be carefully planned on accurately mounted casts, so that results may be visualized prior to the adjustment in the patient's mouth.

• When the first centric relation contact coincides with cusp tips or falls beyond the external limits of supporting cusps *(red areas)*, a centric occlusal adjustment is not workable. Any attempt to continue with the adjustment would endanger the occlusal stability when masticatory forces are directed along the axes of posterior teeth. The manifestation of this problem will be more detectable in the presence of long slide in centric (more than 2 mm), especially when there is a pronounced discrepancy between the configuration of opposing arches and/or great deviation of the transverse hinge axis.

The analysis of centric interferences will define indications and contraindications only for a slide-in-centric adjustment. For example, if a patient has interferences to other functional eccentric movements, occlusal adjustment may be planned to eliminate these interferences regardless of what is dictated by the centric analysis of the occlusal sectors.

Mechanical analogies may be applied to help the clinician make the proper decision about where to adjust. The operator should first conceptualize the teeth as a hammer and an anvil (Fig 8-22). Supporting cusps or any other cusps contacting in maximum intercuspation should be compared to the hammer. Areas of the teeth contacted by supporting cusps correspond to the anvil. When this mental image is employed, the routine to be remembered is always to adjust the anvil and never the hammer. This aids in maintaining centric stops.

The routine that follows describes where to grind on the occlusal surface and explains the dissimilarities between areas to adjust in the maxillary and mandibular teeth. According to the contact relationships explained earlier, proper adjustment of the occlusal surfaces, represented as the anvil on the maxillary teeth, will produce distally oriented stops for the mandibular supporting cusps (Fig 8-23). Accurate adjustment of the mandibular teeth will supply mesially oriented stops for the maxillary supporting cusps (Fig 8-24).

Adjustment for centric relation prematurities on maxillary teeth is commonly performed on inclines, which face mesially. Reduction of prematurities on mandibular teeth is done on inclines that face distally. If extensive grinding is predicted, which may endanger the stability of supporting cusps, grinding teeth on both arches is considered a sound procedure (Fig 8-25).

Color coding

During the occlusal analysis of the casts, it is necessary to use a substance capable of marking the prematurities. In general, articulating paper or ribbon in different colors (usually green, red, or blue) is the material of choice.

If centric stops are marked in red and centric relation prematurities are marked in green, it is possible for the resulting marks to overlap each other at the level of maximum intercuspation (Fig 8-26). Therefore, in addition to the rules already

Fig 8-22 Hammer and anvil concept. Supporting cusps or any cusps contacting in maximum intercuspation are likened to a hammer; areas of the teeth that are contacted by the supporting cusps are considered to be like an anvil. Adjustments should be made to areas contacted by the supporting cusps (the anvil) and not to the supporting cusps themselves (the hammer).

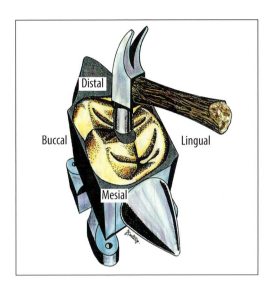

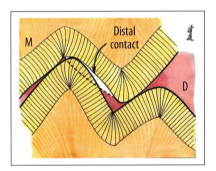

Fig 8-23 Section of two opposing occlusal thirds showing the adjustment for a distal (D) stop. (M) Mesial.

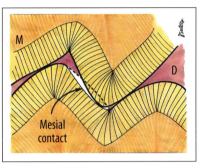

Fig 8-24 Section of two opposing occlusal thirds showing the adjustment for a mesial (M) stop. (D) Distal.

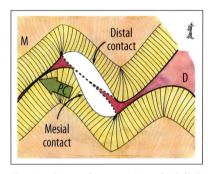

Fig 8-25 Section of two opposing occlusal thirds showing simultaneous adjustment for mesial (M) and distal (D) stops. (PC) Posterior centric stop.

Fig 8-26 Overlapping of marks in maximum intercuspation *(red dot)* and centric relation contacts *(green dot)* on the occlusal surface of a mandibular molar.

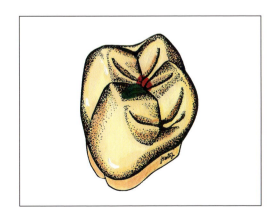

mentioned, when the marks produced on the occlusal surface of maxillary teeth are observed, the red marks will face mesially; on mandibular teeth, these marks will face distally. This guide aids the operator to conceive where the mesial or distal supporting area will follow and to decide where to avoid grinding. In this case, the norm is always to grind the green marks and never the red marks, because adjustments are made in centric relation and not in maximum intercuspation. This practice also helps to distinguish the many spots that occur on teeth during the course of an adjustment.

Eccentric positions

The most significant advice for adjustment in excursive movements is merely to eliminate any interference to smooth gliding movements without threatening the adjustment in centric. It is relevant to consider eccentric adjustment as consistently adjusting interferences in the pathway of movement.

Balancing excursion interferences

For balancing excursions, the adjustment is started on the maxillary teeth, especially those prematurities that are in the way of mandibular movement.

Working excursion interferences

The application of the "buccal of upper and lingual of lower" (BULL) rule is a norm that is only indicated for this type of movement. When the movement of the jaws to the working side is hampered, the adjustment is indicated. The approach is to reduce the occlusal inclines of buccal cusps of maxillary teeth and/or lingual cusps of mandibular teeth.

Protrusive excursion interferences

For protrusive interferences, the nonsupporting cusps are invariably adjusted. In specific situations, if massive protrusive interferences occur on anterior teeth, the adjustment will be limited to the maxillary teeth.

Adjustment techniques

There are definite dental areas that are rarely ground during an occlusal adjustment. These areas include the axial surfaces or any part of the tooth outside the limits of the occlusal table. The procedure should always be stopped if there is imminent probability of dental mutilation.

Centric adjustment

The selection of colors used to mark occlusal contacts is not consequential. For example, green ribbon could be used for centric relation and red for maximum intercuspation.

Maximum intercuspation

The opposing casts are carefully tapped in intercuspal position, and the centric contacts are marked first. If necessary, these marks can be mapped on an appropriate chart. If heavy contacts (bull's eye marks) are detected in this position, judicious relief or rounding of these areas is carried out, but care must be taken to not remove centric stops.

Centric relation

The articulator is now moved in centric relation position. With the condylar elements resting against the posterior wall of the condylar housing, the first contact in centric relation is checked. Some instruments have provisions to lock the condylar spheres in this position. If so, the condylar elements should be locked. In this condition, the casts will now be related in centric relation. With the green ribbon interposed between the occlusal surfaces, the teeth are tapped together gently. Strong tapping at this point could result in passing or missing of the first contacts (prematurities). Next, if the condylar elements are locked, the instrument is unlocked, and the instrument is moved to maximum intercuspation. With the green ribbon interposed between cast, marks will be produced to demonstrate the path of the slide in centric on the inclines.

These premature contacts are removed with the sharp blade of a cleoid or discoid instrument. Small amounts of tooth structure should be removed (further amounts can always be reduced later). It is always a good idea to highlight the areas ground with an orange permanent marker. The use of orange is preferable because it does not obscure any further red or green marks that may be produced later.

Contacts in centric relation are marked and removed continuously to reach the objectives of freedom in centric. A platform will be created at the depth of the occlusal fossa to supply a centric stop for the opposing supporting cusp. The occlusal load in this case will be directed through the long axis of the teeth (Fig 8-27). This goal can be described as the elimination of the vertical component of the slide in centric, where the vertical dimension of occlusion at centric relation is the same as the vertical dimension of occlusion in maximum intercuspation. Marks will shift from side to side and from tooth to tooth during the progression of the adjustment. The maintenance or elimination of the slide is the indicator as to whether the objective of the vertical dimension is achieved.

The best way to monitor the success of this goal is to observe how closely the incisal pin is approximating the incisal table. When the slide disappears, or if the pin is already in contact with the incisal table, the adjustment should be terminated. If

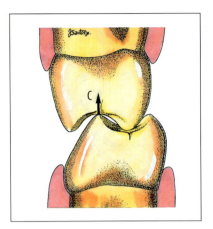

Fig 8-27 Freedom-in-centric adjustment showing the longitudinal direction *(arrow)* of the occlusal load (C).

the procedure is not ended, there is a strong possibility of overgrinding. It is not required to have a centric relation contact for every centric stop in maximum intercuspation, but it is acceptable to have multiple bilateral centric relation contacts and no slide. Figure 8-28 shows an example of a centric relation adjustment that was achieved between opposing left quadrants. Centric relation contacts on anterior teeth are not required or desirable. If they occur, it is an indication of overgrinding.

Eccentric adjustment

Eccentric excursions may be adjusted as required. Articulating ribbons of different colors are utilized for marking. The articulator is moved into definite eccentric movements one at a time. The marks are detected and entered on an appropriate chart.

Balancing adjustments

Once the decision to proceed has been made, all balancing interferences should be eliminated, if reasonable. In the majority of cases, grinding starts on the maxillary teeth. If the tooth being adjusted for balancing excursion has multiple centric stops, it is permissible to remove a stop to guarantee removal of the interference. The balancing side should always be checked after the removal of working interferences. Figure 8-29 demonstrates an example of balancing adjustment on opposing left quadrants.

Working adjustments

Working adjustments are made on occlusal inclines of nonsupporting cusps. The operator should remove small amounts of tooth substance, mark again, and grind

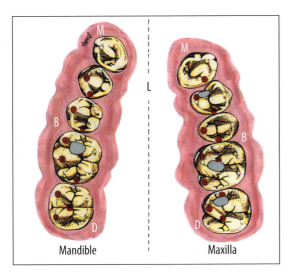

Fig 8-28 Selective adjustment of the posterior teeth in centric relation. No adjustment should be made to the portions of the occlusal surface close to the cusp tips *(red dots)*. The correct grinding *(light blue areas)* represents the areas reduced in centric relation (distal stop for the mandible supporting cusp and mesial stop for the maxillary teeth). This example of centric adjustment was carried out on left opposing arches as represented in Fig 8-8. (D) Distal; (M) mesial; (B) buccal; (L) lingual.

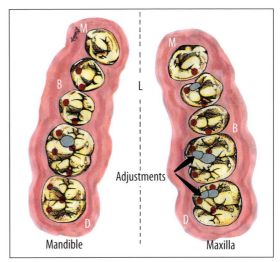

Fig 8-29 Balancing adjustment of the example presented in Fig 8-12. This adjustment was done before the working adjustment. Adjustments *(light blue areas)* were performed mainly in the maxillary arch. The centric stops *(red dots)* were preserved. (D) Distal; (M) mesial; (B) buccal; (L) lingual.

until the desired results are obtained. When the articulator is moved to working relations and group function is detected (Fig 8-30), the elimination of working interferences on the lingual cusps can be carried out. In Fig 8-31, working interferences on left opposing quadrants were removed according to the BULL technique.

When the patient presents canine-guided occlusion for working excursions (Fig 8-32), good judgment must be exercised in the evaluation of the steepness of the anterior guidance. In some clinical cases, a steep guidance must be reduced to provide freedom for eccentric movements.

Protrusive adjustments

Posterior or anterior teeth may be involved in protrusive interferences. Usually, protrusive interferences are found on posterior teeth because any protrusive contact on a posterior tooth is considered interference. When tooth structure is removed from interfering teeth, centric stability must not be disrupted. Figure 8-33 provides an example of the elimination of interferences on posterior teeth of left opposing quadrants.

If anterior teeth need adjustment in protrusion, tooth structure is eliminated from maxillary teeth (Fig 8-34). In the normal arrangement of teeth, the incisal edges of mandibular teeth represent supporting cusps.

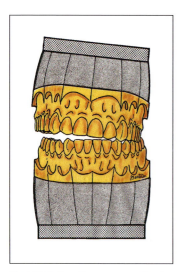

Fig 8-30 Left working movement showing group function as observed on mounted casts.

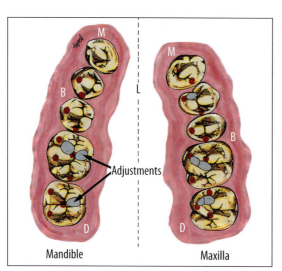

Fig 8-31 Adjustments *(light blue areas)* of the example in Fig 8-15 to eliminate working interference. This working adjustment may follow the balancing adjustment. In accordance with the BULL technique (buccal cusps of upper teeth; lingual cusps of lower teeth), only the lingual inclines of the mandibular molars were adjusted to eliminate a cross-tooth balance. Centric stops *(red dots)* were preserved. (D) Distal; (M) mesial; (B) buccal; (L) lingual.

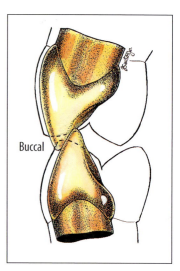

Fig 8-32 Canine-guided relationship.

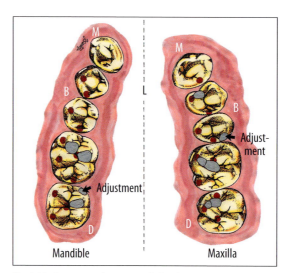

Fig 8-33 Protrusive adjustments *(light blue areas)* of the interferences represented in Fig 8-16. Just the cusp arms of the maxillary second premolar and second molar were adjusted. The centric stops *(red dots)* as well as the anterior protrusive guidance were preserved. (D) Distal; (M) mesial; (B) buccal; (L) lingual.

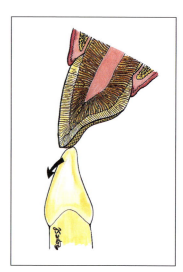

Fig 8-34 Adjustment of incisors (in this case a central incisor) for protrusive movement *(arrow)*.

OCCLUSAL ADJUSTMENT IN THE MOUTH

When the adjustment has been completed as planned on mounted casts, all ground areas should be highlighted with the permanent marker. It is also important to transfer, to an appropriate chart, indications of the occlusal surfaces that were ground during the adjustment. The professional may easily explain to the patient what is going to be done in the mouth with the aid of this visual display. Moreover, sequences of occlusal adjustment will be substantially simplified when the professional has a discernible image of the adjustment on casts.

Before any portion of the occlusal surface is ground, it is important to mark first centric occlusion contacts in the patient's mouth. The patient should tap the teeth together on articulating ribbon or paper (red, preferably). These contacts must be scrupulously respected during the grinding process.

Principles of freedom in centric grant great latitude when areas of the tooth are being ground. Provided that no reduction of critical centric stops is occurring, grinding on inclines may be carried out to duplicate in the patient's mouth the actions performed on the casts. After completion of the adjustment, there should be no slide in centric and no interferences. The ground areas should be well polished to complete the procedure.

OCCLUSION OVER IMPLANTS

In recent years, the interest in osseointegrated implants has grown considerably. Little is known about the occlusal scheme that must be developed over implants.[8–11] Normally, the concepts used for the natural dentition and edentulous conditions have been advocated for adjusting and creating occlusal patterns that might be compatible with implant dentition. However, implants (which are composed of abutment and fixtures) are osseointegrated to bone, producing a sort of "ankylosis" at the basal structure. In contrast to natural teeth, these implants are relatively immobile. This situation creates a need for axial loading of the implants. Horizontal components of force during chewing are to be avoided, because horizontal stresses applied to implant elements may cause damage or bone resorption around fixtures.

The need to plan the adjustment of the occlusion over implants, according to the concepts of freedom in centric, will be discussed in this section. Freedom in centric has been demonstrated to be compatible with axial loading of the dentition.[8–11]

During the planning phase for the insertion of single or multiple implants, in one or both sides of either dental arch, provisions must be made to orient the

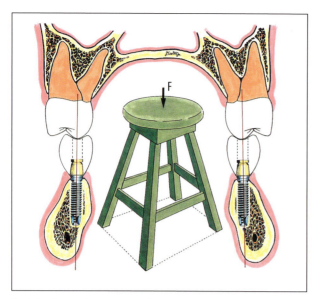

Fig 8-35 Force polygon concept of resultant forces (F) over implants.

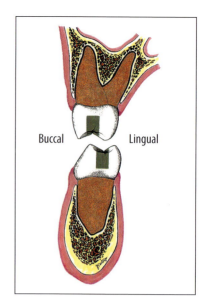

Buccal   Lingual

Fig 8-36 Area of freedom in centric *(green area)* on the central fossa of opposing molars.

total masticatory force according to the force polygon principle (Fig 8-35). The orientation of the long axis of the fixtures (on the frontal and sagittal views) must be compatible with occluding elements to generate masticatory forces that are practically parallel to each other. Any deviation from this norm will tend to create components of horizontal forces, which may be detrimental to the stability of the implants.

Similar to what occurs in the natural dentition, the planning and/or adjustment of the occlusion according to the freedom-in-centric concept must create centric platforms in the range of 2 to 3 mm for opposing supporting cusps (Fig 8-36). Therefore, any contact over an implant element must be adjusted according to this parameter.

If a single implant is positioned in the arch, the supporting cusp of the opposing tooth must contact the element as closely as possible to the axial center of the abutment of the crown. Although adjacent natural teeth may present several centric contacts in maximum intercuspation, the occlusal surface of the implant must be contoured or adjusted to receive only one centric stop (Fig 8-37). If the abutment of the implant crown is mesially or distally located in relation to its mesiodistal dimension, the opposing supporting cusp must make one contact on the occlusal surface of the crown in line with the axial alignment of the implant (Fig 8-38).

During lateral and protrusive functional movements, all other anatomic occlusal components of the implant crown must clear the crown during eccentric movements of the mandible. For example, for an implant in the mandibular molar area, the only

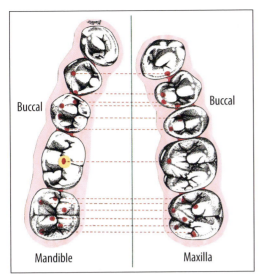

Fig 8-37 Left quadrants of the natural dentition depicting the maximum intercuspation marks produced by occlusal contacts on opposing teeth *(red dots)* and the implant crown *(yellow and red dot)*.

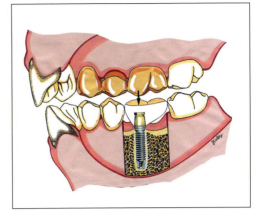

Fig 8-38 Single implant and its relationship with the opposing tooth in centric contact *(arrow)*.

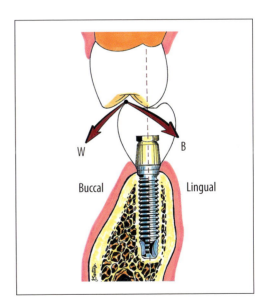

Fig 8-39 Implant inserted in the mandible with the crown in place. Note the freedom of eccentric movement in working (W) and balancing (B) movements. Only centric contact is preserved on the opposing supporting cusp.

contact it should receive would be the centric stop on the depth of the central fossa, in conjunction with the long axis of the implant. Buccal and lingual cusps are shortened to avoid any gliding action against the opposing tooth during lateral working and protrusive movements of the mandible (Fig 8-39). All balancing contacts must be eliminated.

REFERENCES

1. Molina OF, dos Santos J Jr, Nelson S, Nowlin T. A clinical study of specific signs and symptoms of CMD in bruxers classified by the degree of severity. Cranio 1999;17:268–279.
2. Hori N, Yuyama N, Sasaguri K, et al. Effects of biting and response of sympathetic nerve system during restraint stress. Bull Kanagawa Dent Coll 2004;32:123–124.
3. Korioth TWP, Hannam AG. Effect of bilateral asymmetric tooth clenching on load distribution at the mandibular condyles. J Prosthet Dent 1990;64:62–73.
4. Molina OF, dos Santos J Jr. The prevalence of some joint disorders in craniomandibular disorder (CMD) and bruxers as compared to CMD nonbruxer patients and controls. Cranio 1999;17: 17–29.
5. Molina OF, dos Santos J Jr, Nelson S, Grossman E. Prevalence of modalities of headaches and bruxism among patients with craniomandibular disorder. Cranio 1997;15:314–325.
6. Burgett F, Ramfjord SP, Nissle RR, Morrison EC, Charbeneau TD, Caffesse RG. A randomized trial of occlusal adjustment in the treatment of periodontitis patients. J Clin Periodontol 1992; 19:381–387.
7. Greene CS. Orthodontics and temporomandibular disorders. Dent Clin North Am 1988;32: 529–539.
8. Morgan MJ, James DF. Force and moment distributions among osseointegrated dental implants. J Biomech 1995;28:1103–1109.
9. Rangert B, Jemt T, Jorneus L. Forces and moments on Brånemark implants. Int J Oral Maxillofac Implants 1989;4:241–247.
10. Richter EJ. In vivo vertical forces on implants. Int J Oral Maxillofac Implants 1995;10:99–107.
11. Wismeijer D, van Waas MA, Kalk W. Factors to consider in selecting an occlusal concept for patients with implants in the edentulous mandible. J Prosthet Dent 1995;74:380–384.

INTERCEPTIVE OCCLUSAL TREATMENT OF MALOCCLUSION

Most descriptions of equilibration and rehabilitation of the natural dentition present examples according to the characteristics of Angle Class I occlusion (Fig 9-1). In these models, considerations commonly are given to descriptions of, for example, crossbites, maxillofacial discrepancies, diastemata, tooth crowding, tooth drifting and extrusion, uneven plane of occlusion, tooth rotation, absence of teeth, and loss of occlusal structures (Fig 9-2). However, other distorted interarch relationships are not usually discussed.

Any deviation from normal occlusion may be described as *malocclusion*, and in these circumstances corrections are related to orthodontic therapy. However, this treatment may not always be strictly necessary. Individuals with good alignment of the dentition may deviate from what may be considered normal occlusion. Instabilities of interocclusal relationships, especially at the posterior teeth, may demand adjustments or improvements to provide good function.

Therefore, the objective of this chapter is to present the most conservative clinical treatment approaches to render occlusal stability to unconventional interocclusal relationships, even involving what might be considered a malocclusion. In these circumstances, there may be the need to plan and possibly to carry out occlusal adjustments and/or restorations. If the patient has no specific complaints about his or her occlusion, no invasive treatment is indicated. It would be better to leave the situation as it is than to institute procedures that may not provide better end results.

It is not the intention in this chapter to discuss more complex procedures, such as orthodontic corrections, comprehensive rehabilitation procedures, and orthognathic surgery. The discussion will be limited to customary approaches for occlusal equilibration, which may be carried out chairside.

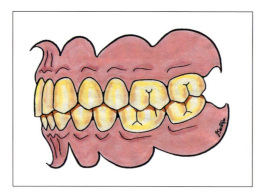

Fig 9-1 Angle Class I malocclusion.

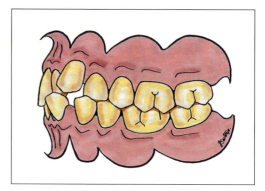

Fig 9-2 Angle Class I malocclusion with distorted relationships.

ARCH CONFIGURATION DISCREPANCIES

It is well known that patients present arches of different configurations. For example, patients may have a triangular maxillary arch (especially those with Angle Class II division 1 malocclusion) and an ovoid mandibular arch (Fig 9-3). Morphologic incongruence such as this may hinder occlusal adjustment in the range between centric relation and maximum intercuspation. The clinician may find that the adjustment of the natural dentition may involve cusp tips of premolars (Fig 9-4). Some cases are so severe that they may preclude any centric adjustment. In this case, the only alternative is to eliminate all interferences to eccentric movements or, if necessary, to plan restorative procedures.

CROSSBITES

Anterior crossbites

Sometimes a maxillary canine or incisor is "locked" behind a mandibular anterior tooth (Fig 9-5). In this case, proper anterior guidance for lateral protrusive movements is hampered by the overlap of opposing incisal borders or cusp tips. This condition is also prone to maintain the mandible in a forward position. If the clinical condition does not display extreme deviations, rounding of selective areas on the incisal border of maxillary and/or mandibular anterior teeth may provide the necessary freedom for the mandible to move into retrusive ranges (Fig 9-6).

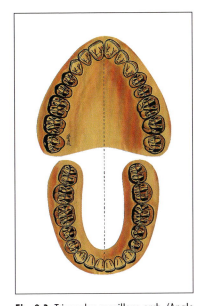

Fig 9-3 Triangular maxillary arch (Angle Class II division 1 malocclusion) and ovoid mandibular arch.

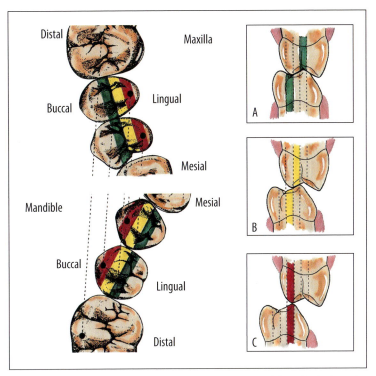

Fig 9-4 Rule of thirds for occlusal adjustment into centric relation. If the occlusal relationship involves contact in the *green areas* (A), no adjustment is needed. If there is contact in the *yellow areas* (B), occlusion may or may not require adjustment. If a patient demonstrates an occlusal relationship involving cusps tips *(red area)* (C), grinding of the cusp tips of premolars may be required.

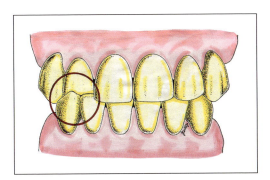

Fig 9-5 Maxillary canine and lateral incisor locked behind the mandibular anterior teeth *(circle)*.

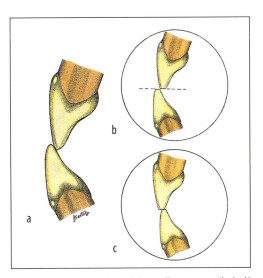

Fig 9-6 Anterior crossbite. *(a)* Maxillary incisor "locked" behind a mandibular incisor; *(b)* rounding of incisal edges of both teeth; *(c)* tendency for correction.

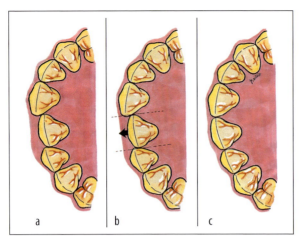

Fig 9-7 Linguoversion. *(a)* Maxillary central incisor kept in linguoversion because of excessive interproximal contour of adjacent teeth; *(b)* careful shaving of interproximal areas of adjacent teeth may provide space for the malpositioned tooth to slide forward *(arrow)*; *(c)* incisor in an acceptable position.

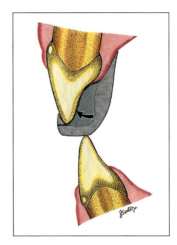

Fig 9-8 Repeated additions of small amounts of quick-curing acrylic resin or light-curing resin composite on the lingual area of a maxillary bite splint. *(arrow)* Direction of the planned labial displacement of the maxillary incisor.

In some cases, a maxillary incisor is in linguoversion because of the excessive interproximal contour of adjacent teeth. Careful shaving of interproximal areas of adjacent teeth may provide space for the malpositioned tooth to slide forward to an acceptable position (Fig 9-7). In this case, it is a good idea to have the patient use a maxillary bite splint for a limited time. The indentation on the appliance at the level of the tooth to be moved must be removed. Small amounts of quick-curing acrylic resin are repeatedly adapted to the lingual area (Fig 9-8). Once the desired movement is achieved, the use of the bite splint is discontinued.

Unilateral posterior crossbites

Unilateral posterior crossbite may encompass total intercuspation in crossbite (Fig 9-9a) or just involvement of cusp tips (Fig 9-9b).

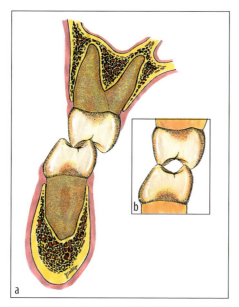

Fig 9-9 Unilateral crossbite. *(a)* Total intercuspation in crossbite; *(b)* involvement of only the cusp tips.

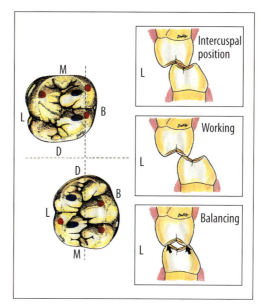

Fig 9-10 Unilateral crossbite. Tendency for interferences on the side of the crossbite with working and balancing eccentric movements. *(blue dots)* Working contacts, which may be reduced; *(red dots)* balancing contacts; (D) distal; (M) mesial; (B) buccal; (L) lingual.

Total intercuspation

In total intercuspation, there is a tendency for eccentric movement interferences on the side of the crossbite (Fig 9-10). Because pointed maxillary buccal cusps and mandibular lingual cusps of posterior teeth are acting as supporting cusps, they cannot provide good stability. Molars will have a tendency to tilt and to produce heavy interferences, especially on the balancing side. If the professional is unable to render immediate orthodontic or restorative treatment, the best approach is to round maxillary lingual and mandibular buccal cusps to attenuate heavy interferences.

If canine guidance is desired, reduction of heavy working contacts may be a good procedure for the institution of an acceptable canine guidance on the affected side. Grinding must be concentrated on the occlusal inclines of both maxillary buccal and mandibular lingual cusps, but care must be taken to avoid eliminating centric stops. Working contacts may be reduced for the purpose of creating canine guidance (see Fig 9-10).

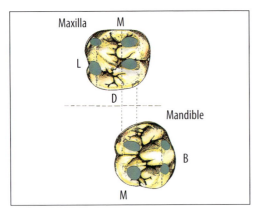

Fig 9-11 Unilateral crossbite. The light blue areas represent the reduction of occlusal inclines of maxillary buccal cusps, occlusal inclines of mandibular lingual cusps, axial contour of buccal mandibular cusps, and axial contour of maxillary lingual cusps to provide sliding ramps to reduce the extent of crossbite. (D) Distal; (M) mesial; (B) buccal; (L) lingual.

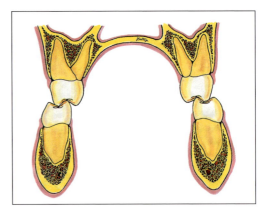

Fig 9-12 Bilateral crossbite. Bilateral relationship of the molars of opposing arches, where it is possible to note the reverse cusp overlapping. The vertical overlap occurs at the expense of mandibular buccal cusps and maxillary lingual cusps.

Involvement of cusp tips

When only cusp tips are involved in crossbite, selective adjustment on some occlusal inclines may produce good results. Reduction of the occlusal inclines of maxillary buccal cusps, occlusal inclines of mandibular lingual cusps, axial contour of buccal mandibular cusps, and axial contour of maxillary lingual cusps may supply sliding ramps to correct the crossbite (Fig 9-11). Care must be taken to avoid excessive reduction of maxillary buccal and mandibular lingual cusp tips to prevent further loss of centric stops and cheek or tongue biting.

Bilateral posterior crossbite

The clinical characteristic of a posterior crossbite is represented by transverse expansion of the mandibular arch involving primarily posterior teeth. Transverse expansion of the mandibular arch may have some implications for centric adjustment. When planning this type of adjustment, the operator must judge if the occlusal relationships involve cusp tips, as explained previously. If so, centric adjustment may not be possible.

Normally, in these cases, anterior maxillary teeth overlap mandibular anterior teeth and, in the majority of the cases, the canines maintain normal relationships. The premolars and molars have reverse overlapping relationships, whereas the vertical overlap occurs at the expense of mandibular buccal cusps and maxillary lingual cusps (Fig 9-12). Readings for movements are totally inverted from the "normal" interocclusal configuration (see Fig 9-10).

Similar to the situation in unilateral crossbite, overlap of cusps may present two forms: in the first, there is only alignment of opposing cusps; in the second, there is total intercuspation. In the first kind of relationship, taking into consideration favorable clinical conditions, the adjustment may follow the same pattern as described earlier for unilateral crossbite (see Fig 9-11). In the second variety, the best approach is to alleviate heavy contacts for excursive movements. Sometimes, the total elimination of interferences is practically impossible.

For both relationships, if clinically feasible, it is possible to create more effective anterior guidance for eccentric movements. Opposing canines may be used to generate canine-guided occlusion for this purpose. The procedure utilizes provisional use of resin composites or laminates applied to the lingual surfaces of the maxillary canines. This treatment supplies immediate guidance for mandibular canines in protrusive and lateral movements. However, it is important to observe if the increase of contour on these areas induces any restriction of movement or locks the mandible in a retruded position. Any amount of change in these areas is critical; therefore, the treatment must be well planned, and periodic supervision of the patient is mandatory.

MANDIBULAR ANTERIOR CROWDING

Crowding of mandibular incisors is one of the most common distortions of the natural dentition. This defect in dental alignment produces several obstacles to the integrity of the anterior portion of dental arches, including the thinning of interproximal alveolar bone, difficulty in cleaning, unsightly localized gingival recession, and an increased risk of periodontal diseases.

Some of the causes of anterior crowding are as follows:

- Deep overbite in Class II division 1 malocclusion
- Reduced transverse distance between maxillary and mandibular canines
- Triangular maxillary arch
- Lack of stable occlusal support on posterior teeth
- Mandibular incisors with narrow crowns
- Class III tendency

If the expansion of the arches through orthodontic procedures presents difficulty, correction may be accomplished directly in the mouth by the use of coronal reshaping. If the mandibular incisors are not tipped lingually, it is possible to generate space for correction by reducing the mesiodistal width of the teeth (Fig 9-13). If the situation is not too severe, rounding of sharp incisal edges and line angles may provide

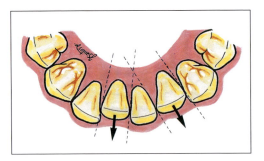

Fig 9-13 Incisor crowding. It is viable to generate space for correction *(arrows)* by reducing the mesiodistal width of the teeth.

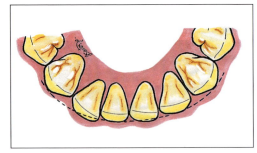

Fig 9-14 Incisor crowding. Rounding of sharp incisal edges and line angles *(dotted line)* provides better interincisor relationships and decreases interferences during functional gliding movements.

better interincisal relationships and reduce interferences during functional gliding movements of the mandible (Fig 9-14).

For the majority of patients, extraction of mandibular incisors may be the treatment of choice. If crowding is not excessive there is no contraindication for the procedure. The only danger is if the treatment causes increased overlap of maxillary over mandibular incisors.

The use of a mandibular bite splint, with regular addition of acrylic resin, may deliver the necessary movement to the teeth. Constant supervision is mandatory. The results may be stabilized with a long-term mandibular bite splint or bonded lingual retainer.

ANTERIOR OPEN BITE

The clinical characteristic of an anterior open bite is an increased space between anterior teeth, making it difficult or impossible for patients to incise food (Fig 9-15). This difficult situation causes many individuals to seek professional help.

In the case shown in Fig 9-15 opposing arches have a reverse curve of Spee, producing a great tendency for heavy intercuspal contacts at the most posterior molars as well as balancing- and working-side interferences. Occasionally some masticatory problems may be associated with this condition, although this is not an indication of a cause-effect relationship.

Although there are several causes for the presence of an anterior open bite, the only reason that will impede any proposed correction is the existence of a

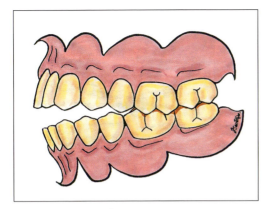

Fig 9-15 Anterior open bite.

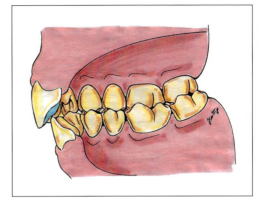

Fig 9-16 Provisional lingual "plateau" *(blue area)* created on the lingual surface of maxillary anterior teeth to provide good anterior guidance and centric support.

degenerative joint disease. Customarily, this condition afflicts elderly individuals. Occlusal bite splint therapy should render relief for the patient in this case.

It is also not advisable to try to increase the vertical dimension of anterior teeth with restorative procedures in an effort to achieve good anterior contacts. This strategy will never be accepted by patients, esthetically or functionally. However, if the patient has a limited amount of anterior open bite, it is possible to create a provisional "plateau" on the lingual surface of the maxillary anterior teeth to provide good anterior guidance and centric supports (Fig 9-16).

If the deviation is not severe, sometimes extraction of third molars may produce substantial improvement.

In the majority of patients, occlusal reductions are necessary. Procedures for adjustment may include judicious grinding of occlusal inclines involved in centric and eccentric contacts (Fig 9-17). Occlusal reduction does not mean destroying the chewing surface of the teeth. Instead of producing flat occlusal tables, the process of adjustment must establish defined occlusal inclines according to the geometric concept (planar representation) presented in Fig 9-18. Before adjustments are attempted directly to the patient's mouth, the sequence of grinding must be well planned on casts mounted on semiadjustable articulators (see chapter 8).

Continuous management is necessary to observe the patient's response to the newly created occlusion and to confirm the maintenance of stable centric stops after the adjustment.

Patients with anterior open bite do not have proficient anterior guidance. Therefore, during the occlusal adjustment for eccentric movements, the only alternative is to preserve some balancing contacts. These contacts will promote posterior guidance for functional lateral movements (medial guidance) to the working side.

If good anterior guidance must be supplied to a maxillary canine, resin composite restorative material or lingual porcelain laminate can be used (Fig 9-19).

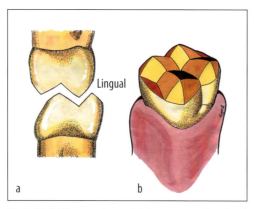

Fig 9-17 *(a)* The posterior vertical dimension can be reduced by judicious grinding of occlusal inclines involved in centric and eccentric contacts. *(b)* Planar representation of a mandibular molar after occlusal reduction.

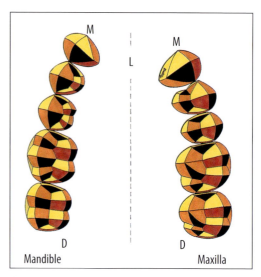

Fig 9-18 Geometric concept (planar representation) of the occlusal surfaces of posterior teeth. (D) Distal; (M) mesial; (B) buccal; (L) lingual.

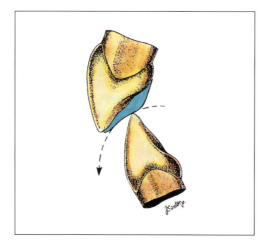

Fig 9-19 Anterior guidance may be supplied to a maxillary canine by resin composite restorative material or a lingual porcelain laminate *(blue area)*.

If porcelain laminate is selected, it is advisable to use a semiadjustable articulator to develop adequate guidance and thickness of the material.

More difficult conditions will demand a combination of invasive procedures, for example extensive reduction of crowns; endodontic treatment; periodontal surgery for crown lengthening; and comprehensive rehabilitation procedures. Considerations about orthognathic surgery or comprehensive orthodontic treatment are beyond the scope of this chapter.

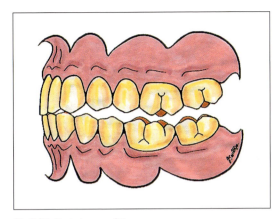

Fig 9-20 Posterior open bite.

POSTERIOR OPEN BITE

Although some individuals may exhibit posterior open bite (Fig 9-20) arising from developmental causes, other patients may develop this problem as part of the aging process or iatrogenically, as the result of prolonged use of some designs of intraoral appliance.

In some instances, the institution of stabilization-type bite splint therapy, with sequential reduction of the vertical dimension of the appliance, may lead to substantial remission of the deviation. However, the recovery of maximum intercuspation is not totally possible.

Because posterior open bites cannot be corrected easily without the institution of complex orthodontic or orthognathic approaches, it is feasible to program the provisional use of porcelain, resin composite, or metallic overlays for patients. The main objective in these cases is to render a stable occlusion. The use of a semiadjustable articulator is an important adjunct to treatment planning.

COLLAPSE OF OCCLUSION

The uneven bilateral position of condyles in the joints may be the result of maxillo-mandibular skeletal malformations during growth or of acute or chronic disorders of the masticatory apparatus. However, the differential diagnosis between these alternatives is very difficult. Both entities have a propensity to present the same response to different modalities of symptomatic therapy. The most obvious detection of the problem, in both cases, is represented by a possible incidence of midline deviation when opposing central incisors are viewed in maximum intercuspation (Fig 9-21).

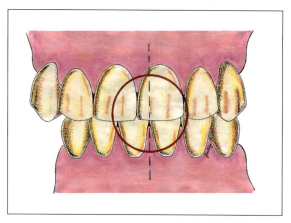

Fig 9-21 Midline deviation when opposing central incisors are in maximum intercuspation (red circle).

If symptomatic treatment is instituted for the patient (eg, occlusal bite splints, medications, or transcutaneous electrical nerve stimulation), dysfunction in the joints and masticatory muscle is likely to subside. Consequently, both condyles tend to assume an even position in the joints. As an outcome of the new positioning of the mandible in relation to the maxilla, unilateral uneven contact of posterior teeth may be noted clinically.

The collapse of occlusion can also be detected when symptomatic treatment is instituted in patients with skeletal deformities. The following sections will discuss some interceptive corrective procedures that may be carried out by the general dental practitioner.

Skeletal malformations

The institution of occlusal bite splint therapy will usually disclose the collapse after several adjustments of the appliance (Fig 9-22). During each visit, it is advisable to observe if the patient is closing on the appliance heavier on one side than on the other; if so, the response is to adjust heavy areas to produce even and stable contacts on the splint. This procedure is known as *differential adjustment*. The finalization of the therapy will occur when the patient does not complain of masticatory pain when biting on the appliance.

When the appliance is removed from the mouth, it is necessary to note if the midline deviation is being corrected and if there is a tendency for unilateral increase of the interocclusal space between arches. The possible tendency for developing

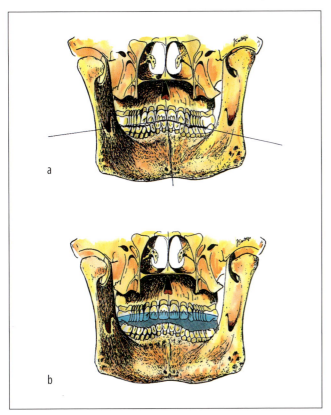

a

b

Fig 9-22 Occlusal bite splint therapy may be able to disclose the collapse of occlusion after several sessions of adjustments of the appliance. *(a)* Eccentric jaw due to collapse of occlusion. *(b)* Condyles centered with the use of a bite splint.

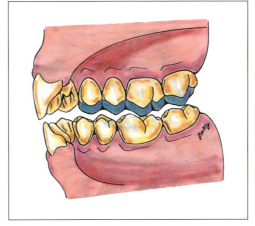

Fig 9-23 Overlay *(blue area)* to provide provisional occlusal stability in collapse of occlusion.

unilateral occlusal clearance may be detected more promptly when the symptomatic treatment is carried out using transcutaneous electronic nerve stimulation.

The use of overlays fabricated with any restorative material may provide provisional occlusal stability. These overlays (Fig 9-23) may be produced directly in the patient's mouth, using a functionally generated path ("chew-in technique"), or on mounted casts.

Grinding of premature contacts on the contralateral side of the arches is not indicated, because it would cause a decrease of vertical dimension and impingement on the anterior teeth.

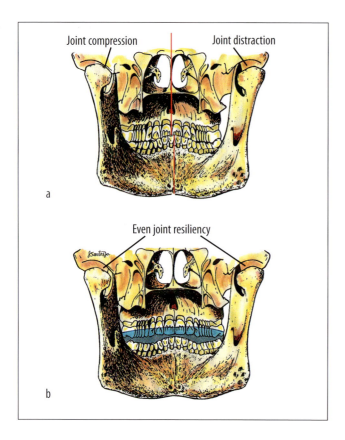

Joint compression   Joint distraction

a

Even joint resiliency

b

Fig 9-24 Distorted position of the mandibular bone because of masticatory muscle imbalances. *(a)* Eccentric jaw due to muscle imbalance. *(b)* Midline correction with bite splint therapy.

Distorted condylar position

Although the mechanisms that cause such deviations are different from those previously described, the outcomes are similar. In this case, the patient may present a distorted position of the mandible, producing different mechanical reactions in the joints (compression and distraction) (Fig 9-24). Midline deviations are more frequently observed in these cases.

Treatment should follow the same pattern as described for skeletal malformations.

CHANGES IN VERTICAL DIMENSION

Loss or increase of the vertical dimension of occlusion is very difficult to determine. Patients are likely to present loss of vertical dimension, and important decisions are constantly necessary to correct the problem.

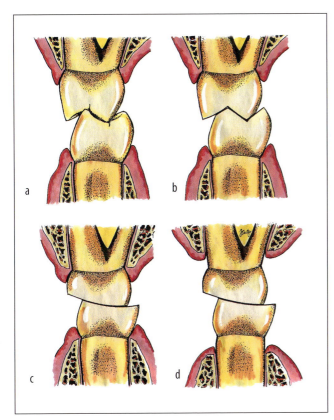

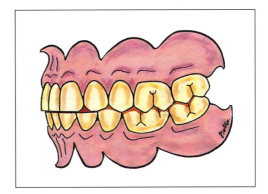

Fig 9-26 Result of anterior bruxism.

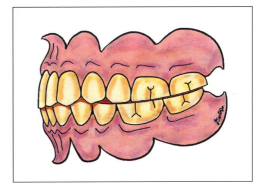

Fig 9-25 Vertical dimension. *(a)* Occlusal relationships of a young individual. *(b)* A constant compensatory extrusion mechanism keeps the maxillomandibular relationships practically stable. *(c)* Loss of vertical dimension that may be the result of an aggressive habit of eccentric bruxism; in this case, the damage may have occurred so rapidly that there was no time for compensatory extrusion. *(d)* Long-term case of eccentric bruxism in which compensatory extrusion has maintained the vertical dimension.

Fig 9-27 Result of posterior bruxism.

The most suggestive type of loss of vertical dimension may be the result of an aggressive habit of eccentric bruxism. Generally, there is no true loss of vertical dimension, because a constant compensatory extrusion mechanism will keep maxillomandibular relations practically stable (Fig 9-25). This phenomenon is easily observed by the extensive reduction of coronal height.

To program an increase of vertical dimension in these circumstances is difficult. The wear of the dentition may occur in segments of dental arches. If the patient exhibits anterior bruxism (Fig 9-26) or posterior bruxism (Fig 9-27), all treatment decisions should include coronal reconstructions of all teeth in both arches. No segmental approach would be acceptable.

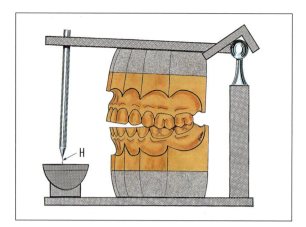 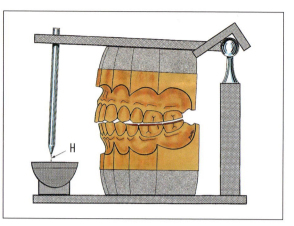

Fig 9-28 If the patient has substantial loss of tooth structure on the anterior portion of both arches because of bruxism, the increase of vertical dimension is questionable. Posterior teeth tend to keep constant vertical relationships. (H) Height of displacement of the incisal pin.

Fig 9-29 Loss of structure of posterior teeth seems to present favorable conditions. An opening of the jaw around an orbiting axis will provide possibilities for an increase of vertical dimension. (H) Height of displacement of the incisal pin.

The amount of necessary bite raising should be assessed with casts mounted in a semiadjustable articulator. If the patient has substantial loss of tooth structure on the anterior portion of the arches, the increase of vertical dimension is questionable, because posterior teeth tend to keep constant vertical relationships (Fig 9-28). Periodontal surgery for coronal elongation would be necessary. The extraction of third molars may help to correct the situation.

Loss of structure of posterior teeth seems to present the most favorable situation. If the patient presents opening of the jaw around an orbiting axis, a modest increase will be acceptable (Fig 9-29). The required amount of vertical dimension increase must be assessed on mounted casts. In addition, periodontal surgery for posterior crown lengthening also must be contemplated.

Likewise, comprehensive restorative procedures and/or selective extractions must be well planned on a semiadjustable articulator. Materials such as porcelain, resin composite, or metallic overlays may be selected in these circumstances. Prescription of continuous use of an occlusal bite splint is essentially mandatory.

ANTERIOR DISPLACEMENT OF THE MANDIBLE

Some patients may acquire anterior open bite as a result of remodeling processes in the joints from temporomandibular disorders or after prolonged use of anterior mandibular repositioning appliances.

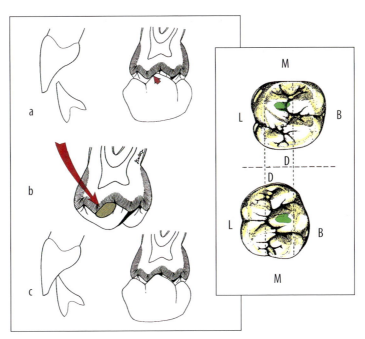

Fig 9-30 Adjustment of the occlusion to an anterior position. *(a)* Before treatment. Grinding will be carried out on the distal cuspal incline of the maxillary tooth *(arrow)*. *(b)* *Arrow* indicates area where selective grinding will be performed. *(inset) Green areas* indicate where grinding will be performed on the inclines. *(c)* After treatment. (D) Distal; (M) mesial; (B) buccal; (L) lingual.

These conditions may demand the adjustment of the occlusion to an anterior position. Preliminary planning for the procedure must be carried out on mounted casts. In general, distal cuspal inclines of maxillary posterior teeth and mesial cuspal inclines of mandibular posterior teeth are involved in this type of adjustment (Fig 9-30).

LOSS OF ANTERIOR GUIDANCE DUE TO PARAFUNCTIONAL HABITS

Consequences of anterior bruxism can account for substantial loss of tooth substance. The most obvious result of this problem is the loss of proper anterior guidance during eccentric movements of the jaw.

Patients with this kind of problem have a tendency to develop posterior guidance for working and protrusive functional movements. If the individual presents group

213

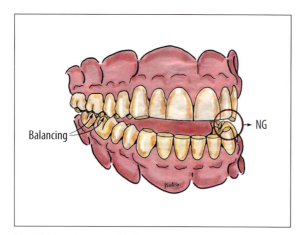

Fig 9-31 Development of balancing-side guidance for working and protrusive movements (medial guidance). (NG) Non-guidance.

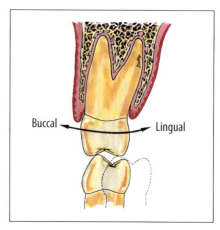

Fig 9-32 Presence of jiggling movement of a maxillary premolar, which is used for working-side guidance.

function during chewing action, the teeth should display heavy contacts on working inclines. If the patients were using their canines to guide excursive movements, the excessive wear of these teeth would produce further deficient guidance. There will be a tendency to develop balancing-side guidance for working and protrusive movements (medial guidance; Fig 9-31).

Eventually, as a result of heavy masticatory loads, it may be possible to detect episodes of trauma from occlusion in areas not normally subject to increased horizontal components. A good example is the presence of "jiggling" movements of one or more premolars, which have started to be used for working-side guidance (Fig 9-32). Teeth involved in this problem may present fremitus that may be clinically detected with digital palpation, when the patient taps the teeth together continually in maximum intercuspation. In extreme cases of trauma from occlusion, this same type of fremitus would be sensed by the examiner when palpating areas where molars are used for medial guidance.

There is little latitude to adjust the occlusion of these patients as far as eccentric mandibular displacements are concerned, especially in cases of medial guidance. The predominant treatment should be to slightly reduce heavy sliding action between inclines and to provide further polishing of occlusal surfaces. For instance, if premolars are involved in working guiding movements, careful reduction of the mesial inclines of maxillary buccal cusps should help to control the problem. This adjustment should improve sliding actions, eliminate fremitus, and, consequently, provide smooth movement between dental surfaces during gliding functional movements. To prevent the recurrence of the problem, it is advisable to prescribe the use of occlusal bite splints.

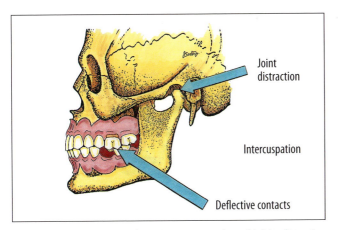

Fig 9-33 Deflective intercuspal position contacts and possibly joint distraction can result.

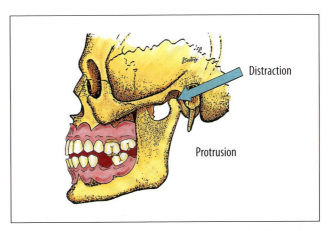

Fig 9-34 Because of interferences in protrusive movement, there is a tendency for joint distraction.

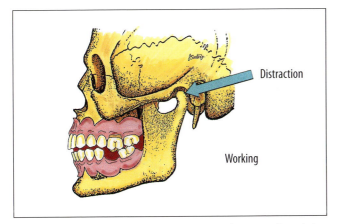

Fig 9-35 Extruded and drifted teeth may also prevent adequate working relationships. There may be potential for mechanical responses in the joints (such as distraction of the joint).

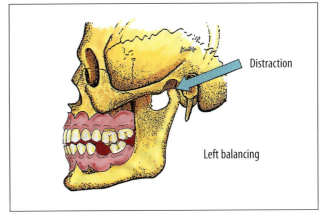

Fig 9-36 A deflective contact on the balancing side, arising from tooth malpositioning, may also increase the potential for mechanical responses in the joints such as distraction).

UNEVEN PLANE OF OCCLUSION

Consistently, corrections of the alignment of the plane of occlusion demand comprehensive and complex rehabilitation procedures. If the deflective contact is too heavy, there will be a tendency for distraction in the ipsilateral temporomandibular joint in the intercuspal position and during excursive movements of the jaw (Figs 9-33 to 9-36). For instance, if the involved teeth are prepared to prosthetically correct the plane of occlusion, the sudden reduction of the vertical dimension

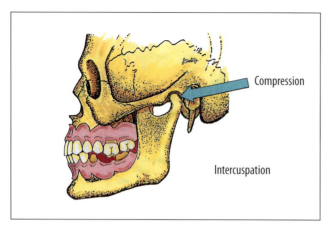

Fig 9-37 When teeth are prepared to prosthetically correct the plane of occlusion, the sudden reduction of the vertical dimension may produce reverse responses on temporomandibular joints. In maximum intercuspation, for example, the tendency will be joint compression.

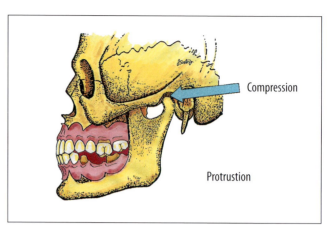

Fig 9-38 Reduction of tooth crown heights may result in ipsilateral joint compression in protrusion.

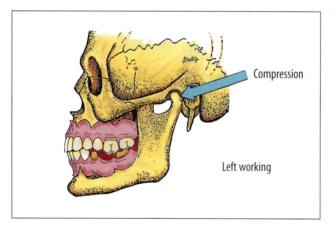

Fig 9-39 The sudden reduction of crown heights result in joint compression in eccentric functional movement to the working side.

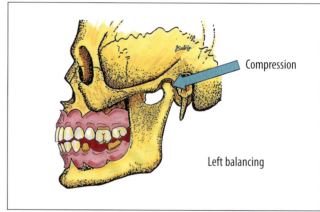

Fig 9-40 Increased compression in the joint during balancing movement may be the result of crown preparation with extensive reduction of cuspal heights.

may produce undesirable responses on the temporomandibular joints. In this case, the reduction of tooth crown heights may cause ipsilateral joint compression in maximum intercuspation and during eccentric functional movements (Figs 9-37 to 9-40).

To prevent unpredictable responses in the joints, it is advisable to capture the proper maxillomandibular relationships on mounted casts on a semiadjustable articulator before any tooth preparation is initiated. Casts should be mounted in centric relation. If there are difficulties in obtaining an occlusal centric relation

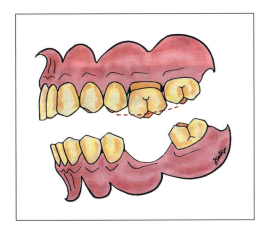

Fig 9-41 A rough reduction of the occlusal overhang *(dotted line)* will improve occlusal relation registrations.

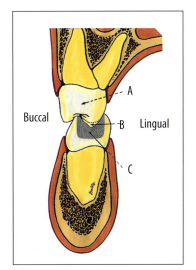

Fig 9-42 Occlusal interferences resulting from restorations with excessively deep fossae. There is overeruption and tilting of the opposing tooth (A). The plane can be corrected through occlusal adjustment and reduction of cuspal height through grinding (B) and placement of new restorations (C).

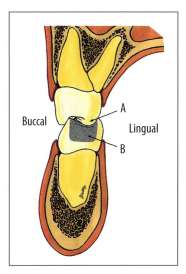

Fig 9-43 The plane of occlusion has been corrected through reshaping of the opposing cusp (A) and restorative procedures (B).

record because of some dysfunctional problem, the institution of provisional bite splint therapy is of great value. In some clinical circumstances, the extrusion of one tooth is very pronounced. In this case, reduction of the occlusal overhang before interocclusal registration is recommended (Fig 9-41).

The utilization of occlusal adjustment and reduction of cuspal height through grinding and placement of new restorations may provide good results in cases of an uneven plane of occlusion (Figs 9-42 and 9-43). However, some teeth are so malpositioned that attainment of an even plane of occlusion would mean substantial reduction of tooth structure and consequent endodontic involvement.

If feasible, vertical reduction of a tooth crown may be carried out with the utilization of systematic grinding of inclines on the occlusal table. With the objective to produce effective chewing results for different groups of teeth, grinding should follow the particular geometric dispositions of the anatomic elements of occlusal surfaces (see Figs 9-17 and 9-18).

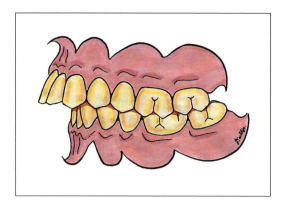

Fig 9-44 Class II division 1 malocclusion.

CLASS II MALOCCLUSION

Division 1

According to the Angle classification, the mandible maintains a disto-occlusal relationship to the maxillary arch in Class II division 1 malocclusion. Mandibular first molars are distally located in relation to maxillary first molars.

Maxillary incisors have a tendency toward labioversion (Fig 9-44). In general, these characteristics are peculiar to patients with this kind of malocclusion; however, other deviations can be detected, such as a triangular maxillary arch, extensive overjet, increased curve of Spee, short mandibular arch, deficient anterior guidance, and a tendency for balancing contacts or medial guidance.

Sometimes, mouth opening is restricted by the small size of the mandible. There is a predominance of protrusive displacement of the jaw, indicating dominant use of this position for chewing.

Because of the incongruence between opposing arches, centric adjustment in the retrusive range of mandibular movement is difficult, because there always will be a tendency for the occlusion to fall in the rule of thirds (see Fig 9-4). The adjustment of posterior teeth to a more anterior position may be a good approach. Grinding of the distal cuspal inclines of maxillary posterior teeth and the mesial cuspal inclines of mandibular posterior teeth may create anterior freedom (Fig 9-45).

If the patient has a tendency for medial guidance (balancing-side guidance) because of a lack of proper anterior guidance, it is not advisable to eliminate balancing contacts. The best approach in this case is to shave all inclines involved in the movement. Further polishing of the occlusal surfaces should render smooth gliding movement to the mandible. This care will prevent any interference with mandibular movement, commonly observed in these situations.

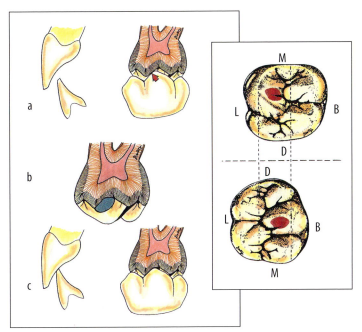

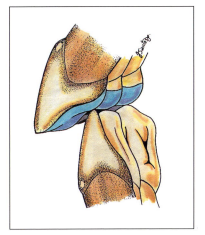

Fig 9-45 Selective grinding to a predetermined anterior position. *(a)* Before treatment. Grinding will be carried out on the distal cuspal incline of the maxillary tooth *(arrow)*. *(b)* Selective grinding will be performed in the *blue area*. *(inset) Red areas* indicate where grinding may be performed. *(c)* After treatment. (D) Distal; (M) mesial; (B) buccal; (L) lingual.

Fig 9-46 Use of resin composite material to create a lingual plateau on maxillary anterior teeth to stabilize occlusal contact relationships.

If the clinical deviation is not too severe, the use of resin composite materials to create a lingual plateau on maxillary anteriors may help to stabilize occlusal contact relationships at this level (Fig 9-46). However, this method only represents a provisional treatment.

Division 2

Class II division 2 malocclusion also presents disto-occlusion of the mandibular arch. In its interocclusal characteristics, it is totally dissimilar from Class II division 1 malocclusion. In Class II division 2 malocclusion, the patient may display pronounced linguoversion of maxillary central incisors, maxillary lateral incisors with

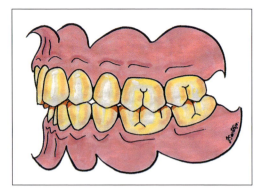

Fig 9-47 Class II division 2 malocclusion.

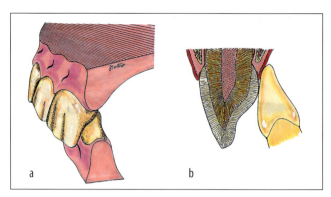

Fig 9-48 Clinical appearance of deep anterior overbite *(a)* and the resulting impingement on soft tissues *(b)*.

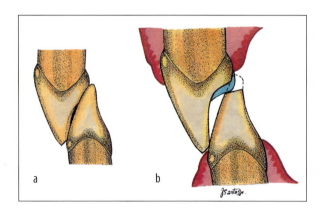

Fig 9-49 *(a)* Deep anterior overbite. *(b)* Reduction of the incisal borders of the mandibular incisors and simultaneous development of a lingual plateau on the maxillary central incisors, using restorative or selective grinding procedures, to produce stable anterior lingual contacts between opposing arches.

labioversion, a U-shaped maxillary arch, no overjet, deep overbite, overeruption of maxillary and mandibular incisors, linguoversion and crowding of mandibular incisors, impingement of palatal soft tissues (especially the incisal papilla), and excessive curvature of the curve of Spee (Fig 9-47).

A tight relationship of the deep overbite may impart dominance of vertical chewing strokes around the transverse axis of mandibular rotation. Because of the small configuration of the mandible, maximum opening may be more restricted than it is in Class I individuals.

This sort of malocclusion has a tendency to self-aggravate because of the lack of occlusal support for mandibular first premolars. Constant wear of the anterior dentition produces thinning of the lingual surface of the maxillary central incisors. The mandibular incisors keep extruding and drifting lingually, producing increased traumatism to palatal soft tissues (Fig 9-48).

Patients with this type of malocclusion have an overt tendency to canine guidance. In general, eccentric movements are well performed and are virtually free of interferences. The only problem is deficiency of stable contacts on the anterior portion of the arches.

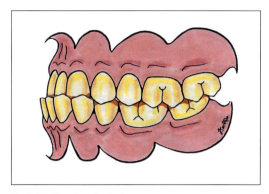

Fig 9-50 Class III malocclusion.

Difficulties involving the treatment of patients with deep overbite lie in problems related to the establishment of stable intercuspal contacts. The main objective in controlling this problem should be the attainment of centric contacts on the anterior portions of the dentition. The use of restorative or selective grinding processes, careful reduction of incisal borders of mandibular anterior teeth, and simultaneous development of a lingual plateau on maxillary central incisors will grant stable anterior lingual contacts between opposing arches. This endeavor may conditionally help to stabilize the occlusion at this level (Fig 9-49).

CLASS III MALOCCLUSION

Patients with Class III malocclusion present disto-occlusion of the maxillary arch. The mandibular first molars are mesially located in relation to maxillary first molars. The curve of Spee is flatter (Fig 9-50). The maxillary arch tends to be narrower than the mandibular arch. All anterior teeth are upright and have a tendency to anterior crossbite. Sometimes distorted vertical overlap at the level of canines and premolars results in diastemata in the mandibular arch. Because of the increased size of the mandible, chewing is predominantly produced around a vertical arch movement.

Posterior contacts are usually unstable, because the trend is a cusp-to-cusp relationship in maximum intercuspation. In the majority of cases, the anterior guidance is deficient, especially concerning protrusive movements.

Because the position of anterior teeth does not provide good anterior guidance, the movement is restricted in this range. The slide from centric relation to maximum intercuspation is very short and has a small vertical component. Chewing strokes around "orbiting" movements are dominant. Presumably, because of the large size of the mandible, opening of the jaw may be more extensive than in Class I patients.

If adjustment is contemplated, it is important to preserve posterior guidance for eccentric jaw movements (medial guidance).

In some cases there is a demand for restorative procedures; therefore, it is important to plan occlusal schemes that will provide stable relationships in centric and good posterior guidance. In some cases, careful planning for third molar extractions may improve anterior relationships for eccentric guidance.

FALSE CLASS III MALOCCLUSION

This type of malocclusion is characterized by the involvement of posterior teeth that force the mandible into a protruded position rather than by a skeletal malformation. In some instances there is no space for maxillary lateral incisors to erupt to a proper position, resulting in mandibular incisors that are positioned labial to the maxillary lateral incisors. This situation also helps to keep the mandible in an anterior position. In general, both arches display compatibly sized proportions; therefore, problems are mostly related to dental positions.

An interceptive treatment for false Class III is the adjustment of posterior teeth to a more retruded jaw position. Reduction of the mesial cuspal inclines of maxillary posterior teeth and the distal cuspal inclines of mandibular posterior teeth should provide the necessary latitude for this position (Fig 9-51). Potential interferences for eccentric movements may preclude the necessary freedom for functional movements of the mandible; hence, elimination of interferences is indicated.

Another modality of adjustment for these cases would be the use of "leaf gauges." Several layers of thin Mylar shims (approximately 60 μm thick) are placed between opposing incisors to produce slight posterior disclusion. Then, one by one, shims are removed until first posterior contacts are achieved. These contacts are ground until anterior contact is again produced on the leaf gauges. Next, one more shim is removed and posterior contacts are reduced again. The process goes on until anterior contacts are obtained without any shim interposed between incisors. This procedure is believed to eliminate most retrusive contacts that have a tendency to protrude the mandible. The presence of mandibular anterior teeth that overlap maxillary incisors may indicate the temporary use of an intraoral mandibular appliance with anterior ramp to guide maxillary incisors to their natural labial position (Fig 9-52).

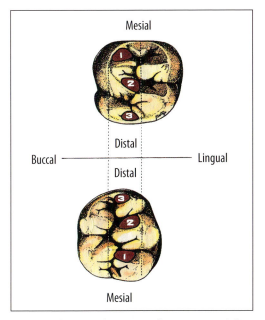

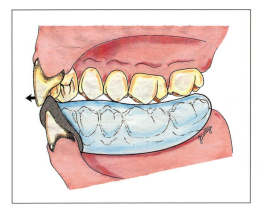

Fig 9-51 Adjustment of posterior teeth to a more retruded jaw position. *(top)* Reduction of mesial cuspal inclines of maxillary posterior teeth (1, 2, and 3) and *(bottom)* distal cuspal inclines of mandibular posterior teeth (1, 2, and 3).

Fig 9-52 Mandibular bite splint with an anterior ramp localized behind the tooth being subjected to labial movement *(arrow)*.

TOOTH MOBILITY DUE TO TRAUMATIC OCCLUSION

It is possible that some teeth that have poor alignment or are subject to direct action of parafunctional habits will become mobile due to trauma from occlusion.

As far as occlusal adjustment is considered, judicious reduction of heavy contacts may be carried out in centric positions. The most practical way to assess these conditions is to employ articulating paper, ribbon, or even thin wax. Some patients usually displays "bull's eye" marks on occlusal surfaces as a result of heavy centric contacts. These marks should be eliminated with rotary instruments and polished later.

The inspection of wear facets produced during eccentric movements may show shiny, wide, flat surfaces that cannot retain good marks when articulating paper, ribbon, or any other marking substance is utilized. It is necessary to relieve these deflecting inclines to improve the slide for eccentric functional movements.

The employment of provisional splinting of teeth using resin composite materials or self-curing acrylic resin directly in the patient's mouth may contribute to management of the problem. If this technique is not desired or indicated, the stabilization-type of occlusal bite splint may be prescribed.

INDEX